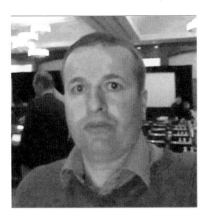

Zviad Gurtskaia. MD. PhD

From the Author:

How to learn Echocardiography? We need to understand the theory, and for that, need to find good book/books. It is necessary to observe and conduct studies. For this, an echocardiography device and a patient are required (not always available). That is why learning Echocardiography last for months. Simulators make things easier but are only available in the university space.

I wanted to create something that would significantly simplify echocardiography learning and teaching. I call it "Echocardiography with simulations" or theory + practice.

The book now in your hands provides the reader with the necessary theoretical knowledge based on the ASE recommendations.

After each chapter, I described how to simulate the Lesson with the online echocardiography simulator MyEchocardiography.com - a powerful online resource that users can use from the comfort of their homes. The many youtube videos from our channel that are linked after each chapter demonstrate the simulation process. The innovative technique significantly reduces the study time and helps to master Echocardiography at the most advanced level.

You can access the Online Echocardiography Simulator when you buy the book. The book comes with a permanent license for the simulator.

Now, it is time Start your Journey in the world of Echocardiography with a new innovative learning methodology ...

I am waiting for your feedback: postmaster@myechocardiography.com

7/23/2023

ECHOCARDIOGRAPHY
WITH SIMULATIONS

Z. Gurtskaia

2023

Table of contents

Table of contents

Let's Start Our Joney in the World of Echocardiography >>>

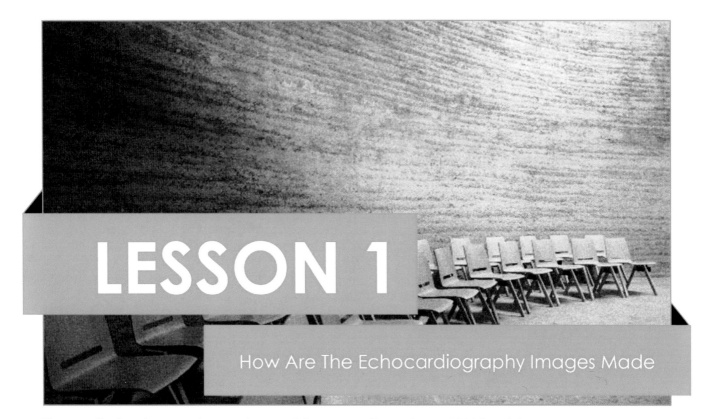

LESSON 1

How Are The Echocardiography Images Made

The patient does not need special preparation for echocardiographic examination; there are no contraindications. The choice of transducer frequency depends on the patient's physique. For obesity, it is better to use a sensor with a low frequency (2-2.5 MHz) because, in this case, it is important to achieve high penetration (depth of ultrasound penetration). In patients with an average build, using a transducer with a frequency of 3.0-3.75 MHz is better. A 5 MHz transducer in pediatrics is often used. In newborns better to use 7 MHz.

High frequency provides high resolution but reduces penetration. In adults, the optimum scanning depth is 16-20 sm. The higher frequency allows you to explore more superficial structures.

Our simulator has a standard frequency of 3.5 MHz.

All cardiac transducers have a small surface that fits easily between the ribs. The transducer has a marker that helps to orient the ultrasonic beam correctly.

The examination can be performed from any position where optimal visualization of cardiac structures is obtained. The patient lies on his left side. The left hand is positioned under the back of the head, which expands the intercostal space, increases the acoustic window, and simplifies examination.

LESSON CONTENT

How Are the Echocardiography Images Made. Echocardiography Views and Positions:

- Left Parasternal View. Long Axis
- Left Parasternal View. Short Axis of the heart at the level of the Aortic Valve.
- Left Parasternal View. Short Axis at the level of the Pulmonary artery
- Left Parasternal View. Short Axis at the level of the Mitral Valve
- Left Parasternal View. Short Axis at the level of the Papillary Muscles
- Left Parasternal View. Short Axis at the level of The Heart Apex
- Apical 4 Chamber View
- Apical 5 Chamber View
- Apical 2 Chamber View
- Apical 3 Chamber View
- Subcostal 4 Chamber View
- Subcostal View of the IVC
- Subcostal View of the Abdominal Aorta
- Suprasternal View. Long Axis of the Aortic Arch

How Are the Echocardiography Images Made

When examining from the suprasternal approach, a pillow is placed under the patient's shoulders, and the head is turned slightly back and to the side to improve visualization.

For user convenience, in our simulation patient is in a vertical position.

The study uses free breathing because deep breathing can distort the echocardiogram.

A special gel is used to improve contact.

In echocardiography, mainly next techniques (Modes) are used:

- Two-dimensional echocardiography (B-Mode)
- One-dimensional echocardiography (M-mode)
- Color Doppler
- Pulse Wave Doppler (PW)
- Continuous Wave Doppler (CW)
- Tissue Doppler (TDI)

User can Simulate all the basic Modes by Echocardiography Online Simulator MyEchocardiography.com

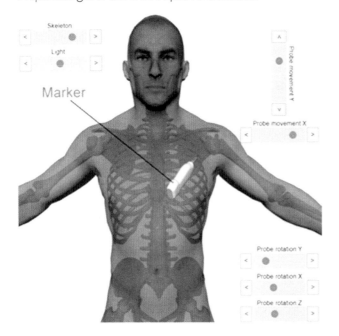

TWO-DIMENSIONAL ECHOCARDIOGRAPHY

B-Mode

Views and Positions

2D Echocardiography

Echocardiography Views And Positions

Two-dimensional echocardiography makes studying heart morphology, pathology, and function possible. However, it significantly depends on the operator's experience and good knowledge of research techniques, hemodynamics, anatomy, physiology, and pathophysiology of the heart.

Many echocardiographic images can be obtained from different approaches. There are several of them (which are the most informative) and are called "Standard Echocardiographic Positions."

It is impossible to obtain a standard position in all patients with the same probe position. The standard position is not the standard position of the transducer - it is the standard image of the heart structures.

- The echocardiographic examination is carried out using the following standard approaches: Left parasternal approach - III-V intercostal space, on the left side of the sternum.
- Apical approach - The transducer is placed in the area of the apical impulse, or somewhat down and The left of it.
- Subcostal approach - The lower region of the xiphoid process.
- Suprasternal Approach - Jugular Fossa.

2D (B-Mode) Examinations

Left Parasternal View:

- Left Parasternal View. Long axis
- Left Parasternal View. Short axis at the level of Ao Valve
- Left Parasternal View. Short axis at the level of Pulmonary Artery
- Left Parasternal View. Short axis at the level of Mitral Valve
- Left Parasternal View. Short axis at the level of Papillary Muscles

Apical View:

- Apical 4 Chamber View
- Apical 5 Chamber View
- Apical 2 Chamber View
- Apical 3 Chamber View

Subcostal View:

- Subcostal 4 Chamber View
- Subcostal View of the Inferior Vena Cava
- Subcostal View of the Abdominal Aorta

Suprasternal View:

- Suprasternal View. Long axis of aortic Arch
- Suprasternal View. Short axis of aortic Arch

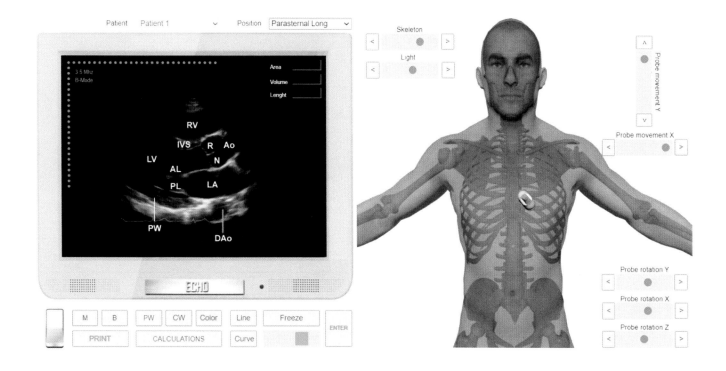

Left Parasternal View

Long Axis of the heart

The transducer is placed in the III-IV or V intercostal space (in our case, in the IV intercostal space) at the left border of the chest bone, perpendicular to the chest surface.

In obese patients, it is better to conduct the study from the III intercostal space; in asthenic patients, it is better to do it from the VI intercostal space.

The transducer marker is pointing up. The heart scan is performed parallel to an imaginary line that connects the right shoulder to the left iliac region - Transducer Marker points toward the right shoulder.

Following heart structures are clearly visualized on the screen:

- **RV** - Right ventricle (Anterior wall and Part of the outflow tract of the right ventricle).
- **IVS** - Upper and middle part of the interventricular septum.
- **AO** - Aorta.
- **LA** - Left Atrium.
- **LV** - Left Ventricle.

- **AL** - Anterior Leaflet of the Mitral Valve.
- **PL** - Posterior Leaflet of the Mitral Valve.
- **R** - Right Coronary Leaflet of the Aortic Valve.
- **N** - Non Coronary Leaflet of the Aortic Valve.
- **PW** - Posterior Wall of the Left Ventricle.
- **Dao** - Descending Aorta.

It is impossible to visualize the apex of the heart from this position because it is slightly lower.

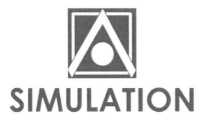

SIMULATION
Left Parasternal View, long axis
Echocardiography Online Simulator
MyEchocardiography.com

- Go to the link https://simulation.myechocardiography.com/

- Run Echocardiography Online Simulator using the **On/Off** Button

- Choose the patient from the list **<<Patient>>** Patient [Patient 1 ⌄]

- Switch Echocardiography Simulator to **B-Mode** [B]   * Initially Simulator is set to B-Mode.

- Using Slider and Buttons **<<Skeleton>>** [<] ● [>]   Choose appropriate transparency level.

- Choose position " **Parasternal Long**" from the List **<<Positions>>** Position [Parasternal Long ⌄]
  or Find the position with the 3D Transducer.

- To change the patient, click the **On/Off** Button

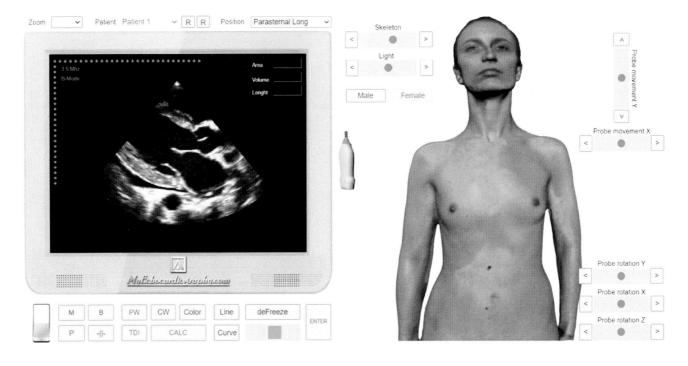

https://www.youtube.com/watch?v=bTH_TF_4XAA&t=8s

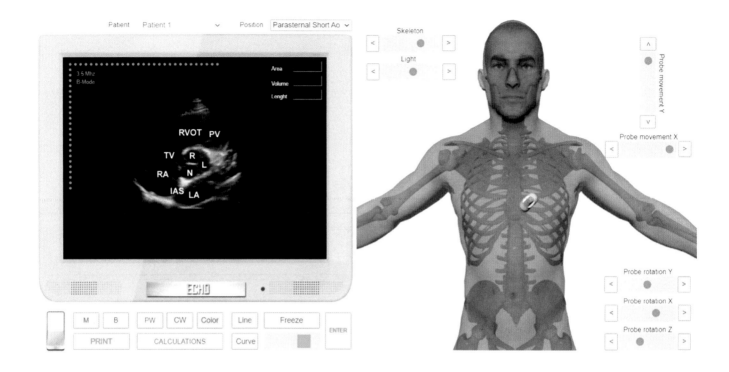

Left Parasternal View

SHORT AXIS AT THE LEVEL OF THE AORTIC VALVE

We must find Left Parasternal View, the long Axis, to obtain this position. Then turn the Transducer 90 degrees clockwise.

The following heart structures are visualized on the screen:

- **RVOT** - Outflow Tract of the Right Ventricle.
- **PV** - Pulmonary Artery Valve.
- **TV** - Tricuspid Valve.
- **RA** - Right Atrium.
- **LA** - Left Atrium.
- **IAS** - Interatrial Septum.
- **R** - Right Coronary Leaflet of the Aortic Valve.
- **N** - Non Coronary Leaflet of the Aortic Valve.
- **L** - Left Coronary Leaflet of the Aortic Valve.

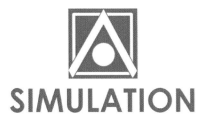

SIMULATION
Left Parasternal View, Short Axis at the Level of the Aortic Valve

Echocardiography Online Simulator
MyEchocardiography.com

- Go to the link https://simulation.myechocardiography.com/

- Run Echocardiography Online Simulator using the **On/Off** Button

- Choose the patient from the list **<<Patient>>** Patient Patient 1

- Switch Echocardiography Simulator to **B-Mode** B * Initially Simulator is set to B-Mode.

- Using Slider and Buttons **<<Skeleton>>** Skeleton < ● > Choose appropriate transparency level.

- Choose position "**Parasternal Short Ao**" from the List **<<Positions>>** Position Parasternal Short Ao
  or Find the position with the 3D Transducer.

- To change the patient, click the **On/Off** Button

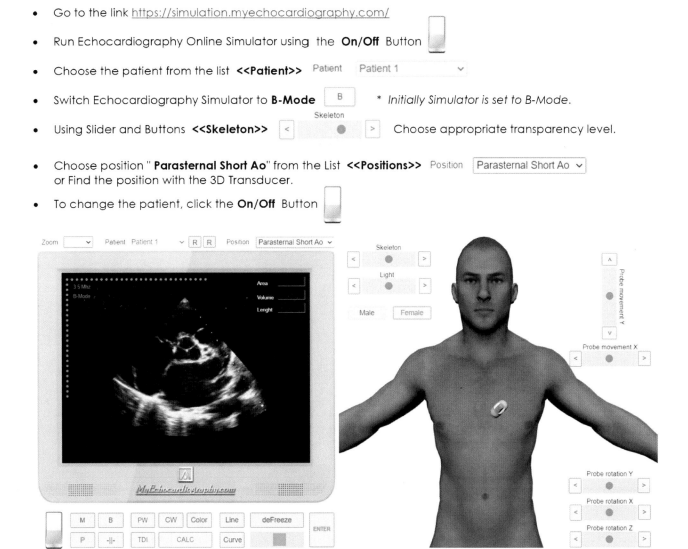

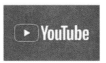

https://www.youtube.com/watch?v=bgBuzFsBfIQ

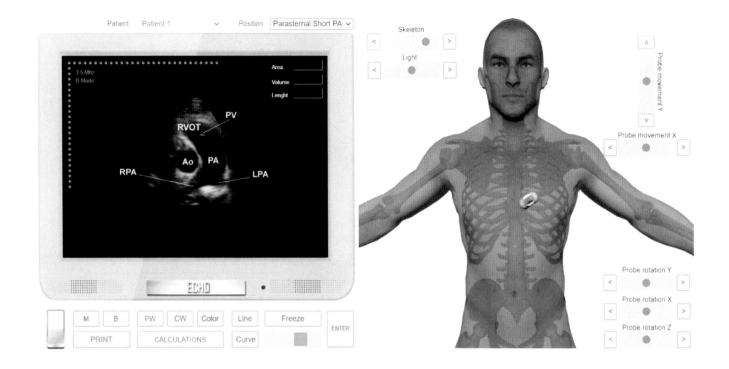

Left Parasternal View

SHORT AXIS OF THE HEART AT THE LEVEL OF THE PULMONARY ARTERY

We must find Left Parasternal View, Short axis at the Level of Aortic Valve. Then slowly rotate Transducer clockwise.

The following heart structures are visualized on the screen:

- **RVOT** - Outflow Tract of the Right Ventricle.
- **PV** - Pulmonary Artery Valve.
- **Ao** - Aorta.
- **PA** - Pulmonary Artery.
- **RPA** - Right Pulmonary Artery.
- **LPA** - Left Pulmonary Artery.

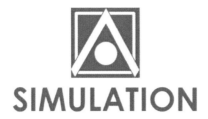

SIMULATION

Left Parasternal View, Short Axis of the Heart at the Level of the Pulmonary Artery

Echocardiography Online Simulator

MyEchocardiography.com

- Go to the link https://simulation.myechocardiography.com/

- Run Echocardiography Online Simulator using the **On/Off** Button

- Choose the patient from the list **<<Patient>>** Patient   Patient 1

- Switch Echocardiography Simulator to **B-Mode**   B   * Initially Simulator is set to B-Mode.

- Using Slider and Buttons **<<Skeleton>>** Skeleton < ● > Choose appropriate transparency level.

- Choose position " **Parasternal Short PA**" from the List **<<Positions>>** Position Parasternal Short PA

  or Find the position with the 3D Transducer.

- To change the patient, click the **On/Off** Button

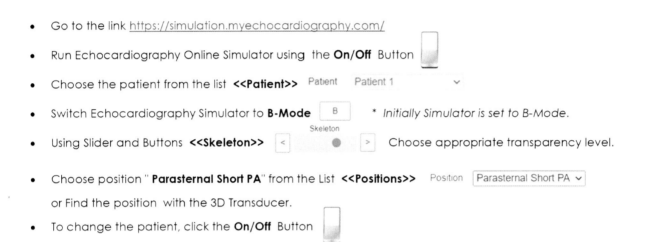

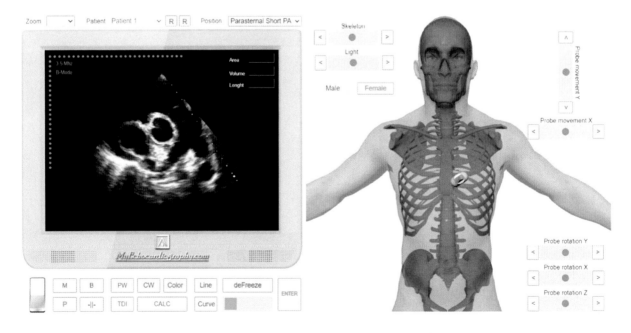

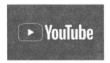

https://studio.youtube.com/video/IBihCY73Zw8/edit

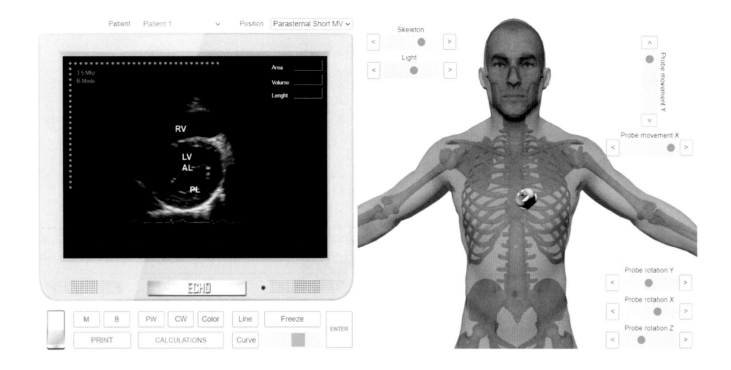

Left Parasternal View

SHORT AXIS AT THE LEVEL OF THE MITRAL VALVE

This position is used to study the left ventricle and mitral valve, for planimetric measurement of the Mitral Valve Area (MVA Tracing).

We must find Left Parasternal View, Short Axis at the level of the Aortic Valve. Then tilt the Transducer a little down.

The following heart structures are visualized on the screen:

- **RV**-Right ventricle.
- **LV**-Left Ventricle.
- **AL**-Anterior Leaflet of the Mitral Valve.
- **PL**-Posterior Leaflet of the Mitral Valve.

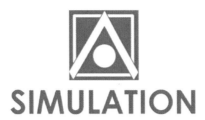

SIMULATION

Left Parasternal View, Short Axis at the Level of the Mitral Valve

Echocardiography Online Simulator

MyEchocardiography.com

- Go to the link https://simulation.myechocardiography.com/
- Run Echocardiography Online Simulator using the **On/Off** Button
- Choose the patient from the list **<<Patient>>** Patient Patient 1 ⌄
- Switch Echocardiography Simulator to **B-Mode** B * Initially Simulator is set to B-Mode.
- Using Slider and Buttons **<<Skeleton>>** Skeleton < ● > Choose appropriate transparency level.
- Choose position " **Parasternal Short MV**" from the List **<<Positions>>** Position Parasternal Short MV ⌄
  or Find the position with the 3D Transducer.
- To change the patient, click the **On/Off** Button

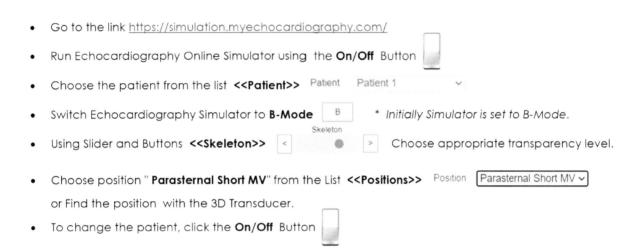

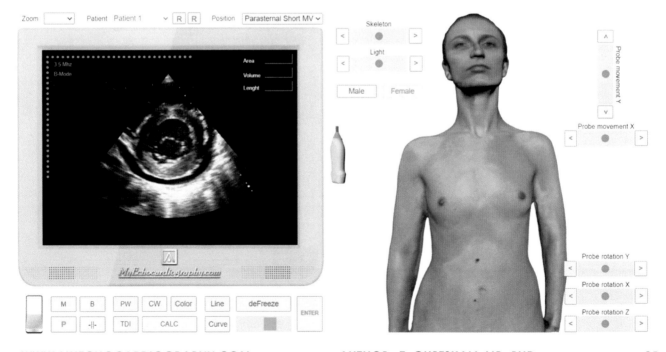

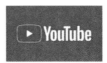

https://www.youtube.com/watch?v=sLZ6g7n5vag

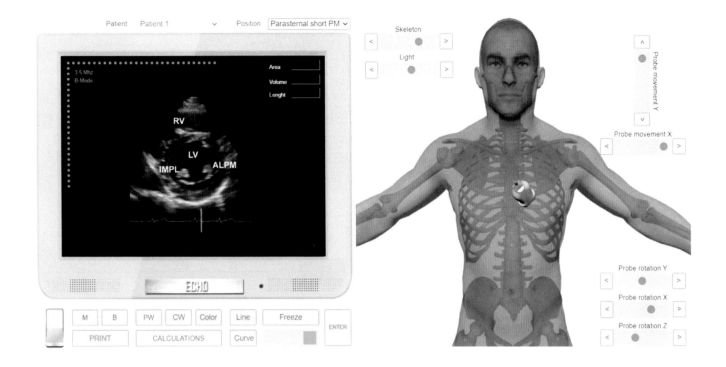

Left Parasternal View

SHORT AXIS AT THE LEVEL OF THE PAPILLARY MUSCLES

This position is used to study the left ventricle and mitral valve for planimetric measurement of the Mitral Valve Area (MVA Tracing).

We must find Left Parasternal View, Short Axis at the level of the Mitral Valve. Then tilt the Transducer a little down.

The following heart structures are visualized on the screen:

- **RV** - Right ventricle.
- **LV** - Left Ventricle.
- **ALPM** - Anterolateral Papillary Muscle.
- **IMPL** - Inferomedial Papillary Muscle.

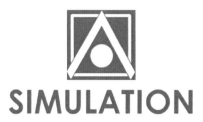

SIMULATION

Left Parasternal View, Short Axis at the Level of the Papillary Muscles

Echocardiography Online Simulator
MyEchocardiography.com

- Go to the link https://simulation.myechocardiography.com/

- Run Echocardiography Online Simulator using the **On/Off** Button

- Choose the patient from the list **<<Patient>>**   Patient   Patient 1   ∨

- Switch Echocardiography Simulator to **B-Mode**   B   * Initially Simulator is set to B-Mode.

- Using Slider and Buttons **<<Skeleton>>**   Skeleton   <   ●   >   Choose appropriate transparency level.

- Choose position " **Parasternal Short PM**" from the List **<<Positions>>**   Position   Parasternal short PM ∨

  or Find the position with the 3D Transducer.

- To change the patient, click the **On/Off** Button

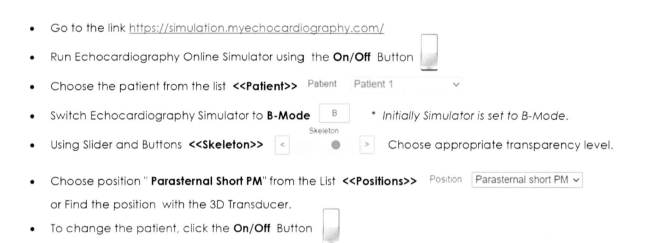

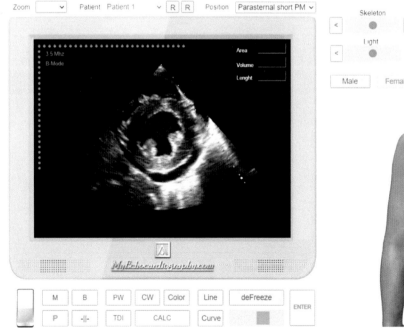

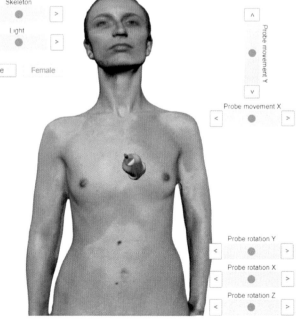

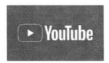

https://www.youtube.com/watch?v=SlrVFhllxJ8&t=10s

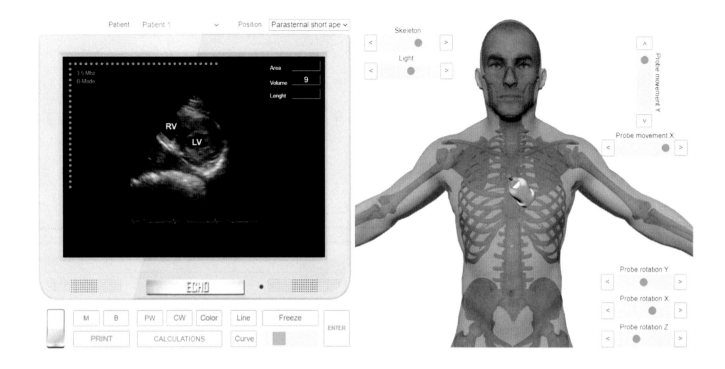

Left Parasternal View

SHORT AXIS AT THE LEVEL OF THE HEART APEX

This position is used to study Heart Apex.

We must find Left Parasternal View, Short Axis at the level of Papillary Muscles. Then tilt the Transducer a little down.

The following heart structures are visualized on the screen:

- **RV** - Right ventricle.
- **LV** - Apex of Left Ventricle.

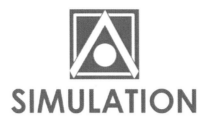

SIMULATION
Left Parasternal View, Short Axis at the Level of the Heart Apex

Echocardiography Online Simulator
MyEchocardiography.com

- Go to the link https://simulation.myechocardiography.com/

- Run Echocardiography Online Simulator using the **On/Off** Button

- Choose the patient from the list **<<Patient>>**   Patient   Patient 1

- Switch Echocardiography Simulator to **B-Mode**   B   * *Initially Simulator is set to B-Mode.*

- Using Slider and Buttons **<<Skeleton>>**   Skeleton   < ● >   Choose appropriate transparency level.

- Choose position "**Parasternal Short Apex**" from the List **<<Positions>>**   Position   Parasternal short ape ⌄
  or Find the position with the 3D Transducer.

- To change the patient, click the **On/Off** Button

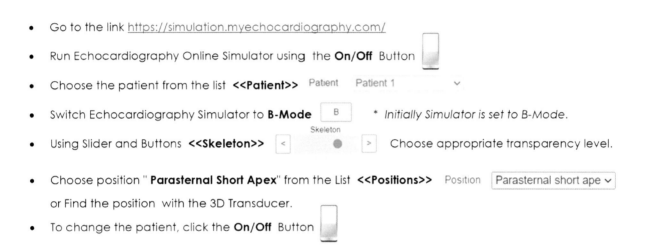

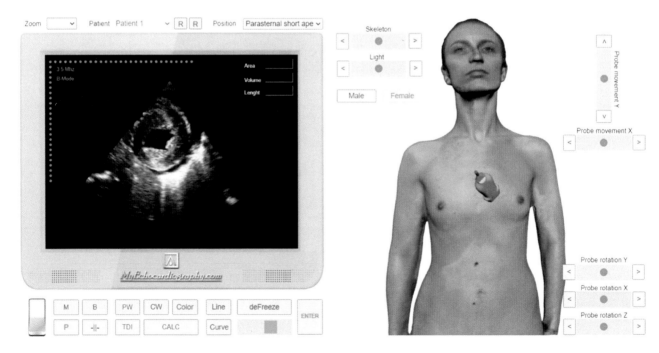

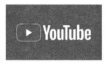

https://www.youtube.com/watch?v=V-MOIXXVO-k

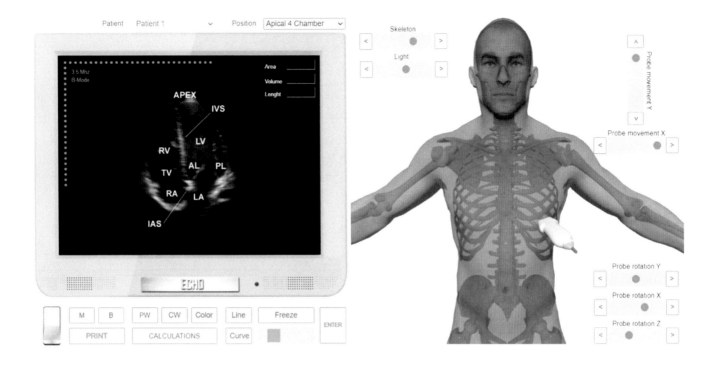

Apical View

APICAL 4 CHAMBER VIEW

Apical 4 Chamber View makes it possible simultaneously examine the left and right ventricles and Atria, atrial and interventricular septum, and mitral and tricuspid valves. Apical 4 Chamber View is one of the best positions for studying local and global contractility of the left ventricle. Only from this position researcher can speak confidently about the dilatation of the right parts of the heart.

To obtain this position Echocardiography Transducer is positioned in the area of the Apex Beat or slightly down and left of it. Transducer Marker is directed to the left (to the right of the researcher). The Central ultrasound beam is directed to the base of the heart (Towards the patient's head).

The following heart structures are visualized on the screen:

- **LA** - Left Atrium.
- **LV** - Left Ventricle.
- **AL** - Anterior Leaflet of the Mitral Valve.
- **PL** - Posterior Leaflet of the Mitral Valve.
- **IVS** - Interventricular Septum.
- **IAS** - Interatrial Septum.
- **RA** - Right Atrium.
- **RV** - Right Ventricle.
- **TV** - Tricuspid Valve.
- **APEX** - Apex of the Heart.

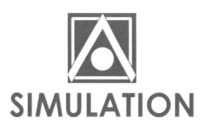

SIMULATION
Apical Four Chamber View
Echocardiography Online Simulator
MyEchocardiography.com

- Go to the link https://simulation.myechocardiography.com/

- Run Echocardiography Online Simulator using the **On/Off** Button

- Choose the patient from the list **<<Patient>>** Patient Patient 1 ∨

- Switch Echocardiography Simulator to **B-Mode** B   * *Initially Simulator is set to B-Mode.*

- Using Slider and Buttons **<<Skeleton>>** < ● >   Choose appropriate transparency level.

- Choose position " **Apical 4 Chamber**" from the List **<<Positions>>** Position Apical 4 Chamber ∨
  or Find the position with the 3D Transducer.

- To change the patient, click the **On/Off** Button

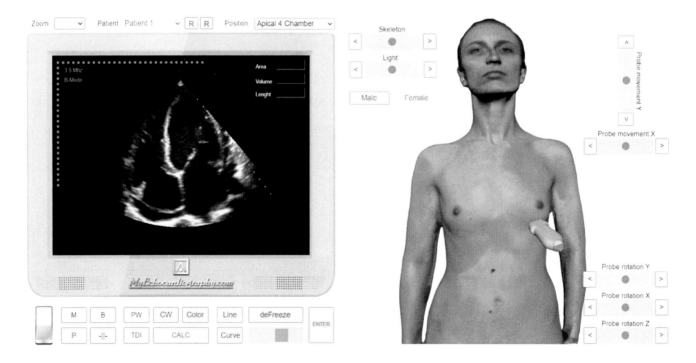

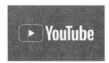

https://www.youtube.com/watch?v=nmuowpqeMEM

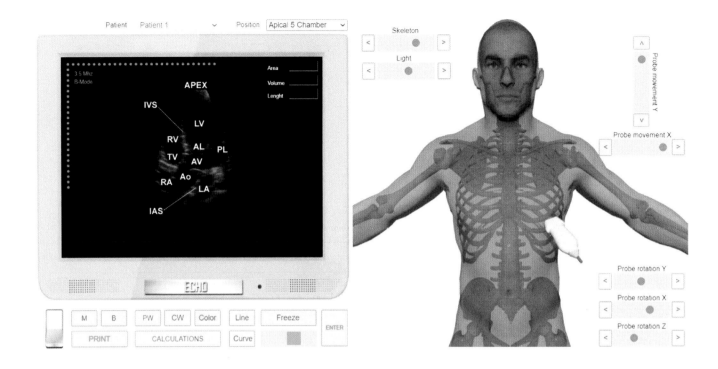

Apical View

APICAL 5 CHAMBER VIEW

Apical 5 Chamber View is the diversity of the Apical 4 Chamber View. It makes it possible to study not only the left and right parts of the heart but also the outflow tract of the left ventricle, the aortic valve, and the ascending aorta (the initial part of the ascending aorta).

The Apical 5 Chamber View is used to study the flow in the outflow tract of the left ventricle and in the ascending aorta with the Color and Spectral Doppler.

We must find Apical 5 Chamber View. The Echocardiography Transducer is positioned in the same way as in the apical four-chamber position, but the Central ultrasonic beam is tilted slightly to the top (See Operations on Transducer). In this case, the ultrasound beam also crosses the ascending part of the aorta.

The following heart structures are visualized on the screen:

- **LA** - Left Atrium.
- **LV** - Left Ventricle.
- **AL** - Anterior Leaflet of the Mitral Valve.
- **PL** - Posterior Leaflet of the Mitral Valve.
- **IVS** - Interventricular Septum.
- **IAS** - Interatrial Septum.
- **RA** - Right Atrium.
- **RV** - Right Ventricle.
- **TV** - Tricuspid Valve.
- **Ao** - Proximal part of the aorta.
- **AV** - Aortic Valve.
- **APEX** - Apex of the Heart.

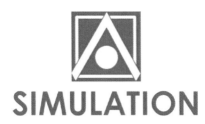

SIMULATION
Apical Five Chamber View
Echocardiography Online Simulator
MyEchocardiography.com

- Go to the link https://simulation.myechocardiography.com/

- Run Echocardiography Online Simulator using the **On/Off** Button

- Choose the patient from the list **<<Patient>>**   Patient   Patient 1   ∨

- Switch Echocardiography Simulator to **B-Mode**   B   * Initially Simulator is set to B-Mode.

- Using Slider and Buttons **<<Skeleton>>**   Skeleton   < ● >   Choose appropriate transparency level.

- Choose position " **Apical 5 Chamber**" from the List **<<Positions>>**   Position   Apical 5 Chamber   ∨
  or Find the position with the 3D Transducer.

- To change the patient, click the **On/Off** Button

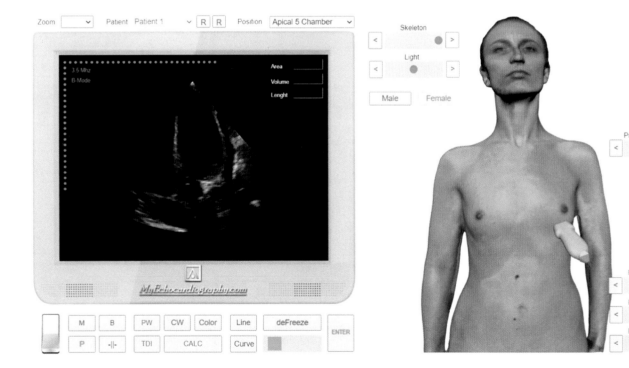

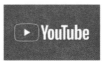

https://www.youtube.com/watch?v=nmuowpqeMEM&t=2s

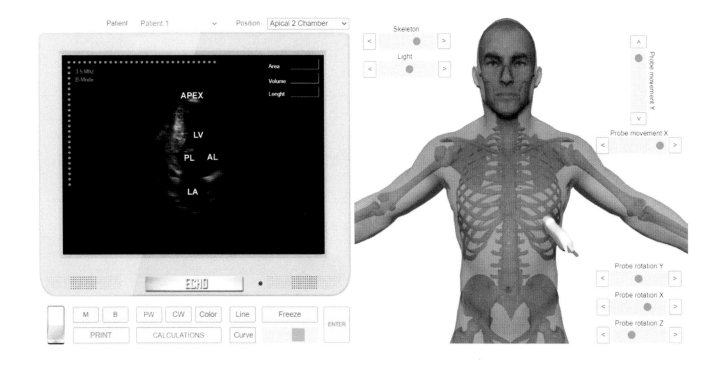

Apical View

APICAL 2 CHAMBER VIEW

Apical 2 Chamber View is used to study the left parts of the heart - the Left Atrium, Left Ventricle, and Mitral Valve. This position is Orthogonal to apical 4 Chamber View

We must find Apical 4 Chamber View. Then Rotate the transducer Clockwise until the right parts of the heart disappear, and only the left ones remain. Sometimes operators have to tilt the ultrasound beam slightly left.

The following heart structures are visualized on the screen:

- **LA** - Left Atrium.
- **LV** - Left Ventricle.
- **AL** - Anterior Leaflet of the Mitral Valve.
- **PL** - Posterior Leaflet of the Mitral Valve.
- **APEX** - Apex of the Heart.

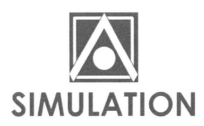

SIMULATION
Apical Two Chamber View
Echocardiography Online Simulator
MyEchocardiography.com

- Go to the link https://simulation.myechocardiography.com/

- Run Echocardiography Online Simulator using the **On/Off** Button

- Choose the patient from the list **<<Patient>>**   Patient   Patient 1 ⌄

- Switch Echocardiography Simulator to **B-Mode**   B   * *Initially Simulator is set to B-Mode.*

- Using Slider and Buttons **<<Skeleton>>**   Skeleton   < ● >   Choose appropriate transparency level.

- Choose position " **Apical 2 Chamber**" from the List **<<Positions>>**   Position   Apical 2 Chamber ⌄

  or Find the position with the 3D Transducer.

- To change the patient, click the **On/Off** Button

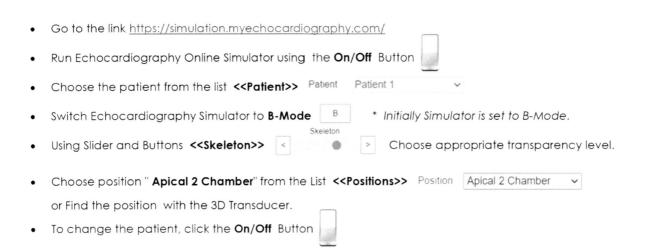

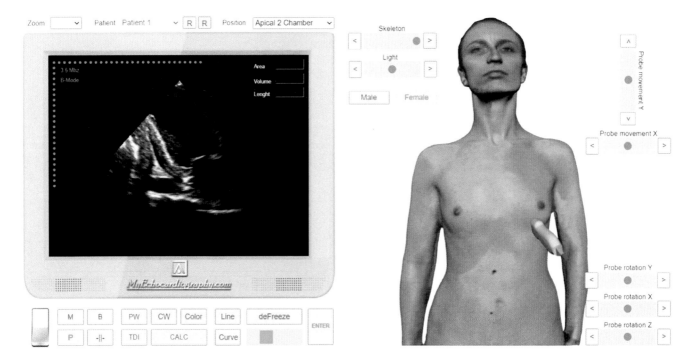

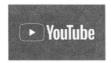

https://www.youtube.com/watch?v=zQUdLLukcoE&t=6s

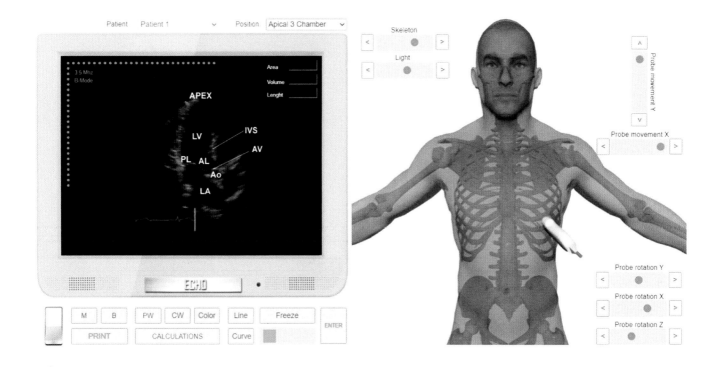

Apical View

APICAL 3 CHAMBER VIEW

Apical 3 Chamber View is mainly used to study the left parts of the heart and Mitral Valve when it is impossible to obtain Left Parasternal View, Long Axis.

We must find Apical 4 Chamber View. Then rotate the transducer clockwise till we see the Apical 3 Chamber View (Sometimes the researcher has to tilt the ultrasound beam slightly left).

The following heart structures are visualized on the screen:

- **LA** - Left Atrium.
- **LV** - Left Ventricle.
- **AL** - Anterior Leaflet of the Mitral Valve.
- **PL** - Posterior Leaflet of the Mitral Valve.
- **Ao** - Proximal part of the aorta.
- **AV** - Aortic Valve.
- **IVS** - Interventricular Septum.
- **APEX** - Apex of the Heart.

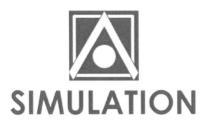

SIMULATION
Apical Three Chamber View
Echocardiography Online Simulator
MyEchocardiography.com

- Go to the link https://simulation.myechocardiography.com/

- Run Echocardiography Online Simulator using the **On/Off** Button

- Choose the patient from the list **<<Patient>>**   Patient   Patient 1

- Switch Echocardiography Simulator to **B-Mode**   B   * Initially Simulator is set to B-Mode.

- Using Slider and Buttons **<<Skeleton>>**   Skeleton   <   >   Choose appropriate transparency level.

- Choose position " **Apical 3 Chamber**" from the List **<<Positions>>**   Position   Apical 3 Chamber
  or Find the position with the 3D Transducer.

- To change the patient, click the **On/Off** Button

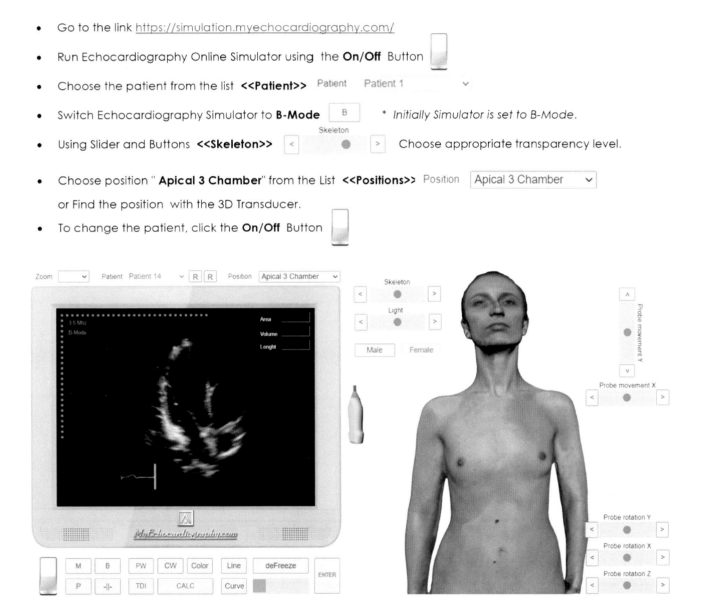

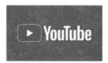

https://www.youtube.com/watch?v=a0tpDXuUTWM

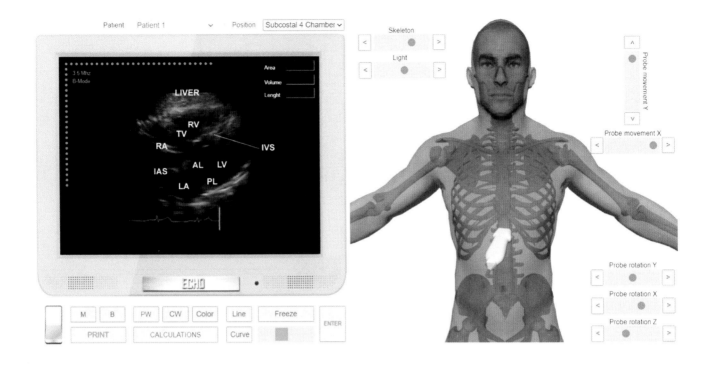

Subcostal View

SUBCOSTAL 4 CHAMBER VIEW

Position the patient supine, with a relaxed abdomen and bent legs if possible. The operator will obtain a good image if a patient stops breathing after inhaling.

Echocardiography Transducer is located 2-3 cm below the xiphoid. The transducer marker is located to the left (to the operator's right). The central ultrasonic beam is directed up and left

The following heart structures are visualized on the screen:

- **LA** - Left Atrium.
- **LV** - Left Ventricle.
- **AL** - Anterior Leaflet of the Mitral Valve.
- **PL** - Posterior Leaflet of the Mitral Valve.
- **IVS** - Interventricular Septum.
- **IAS** - Interatrial Septum.
- **RA** - Right Atrium.
- **RV** - Right Ventricle.
- **TV** - Tricuspid Valve.

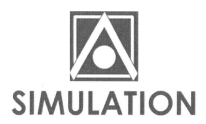

SIMULATION
Subcostal Four Chamber View
Echocardiography Online Simulator
MyEchocardiography.com

- Go to the link https://simulation.myechocardiography.com/

- Run Echocardiography Online Simulator using the **On/Off** Button

- Choose the patient from the list **<<Patient>>** Patient   Patient 1 ⌄

- Switch Echocardiography Simulator to **B-Mode**   B   * *Initially Simulator is set to B-Mode.*

- Using Slider and Buttons **<<Skeleton>>**   <   ●   >   Choose appropriate transparency level.

- Choose position " **Subcostal 4 Chamber**" from the List **<<Positions>>** Position   Subcostal 4 Chamber ⌄
  or Find the position with the 3D Transducer.

- To change the patient, click the **On/Off** Button

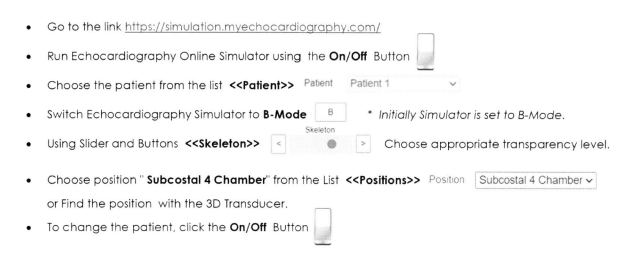

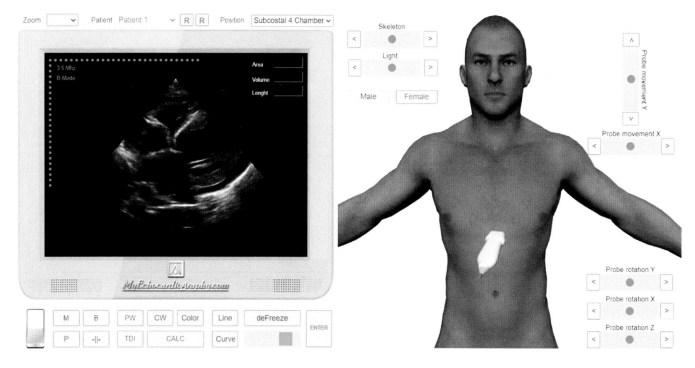

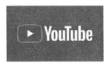

https://youtu.be/9deh8MUkGIU

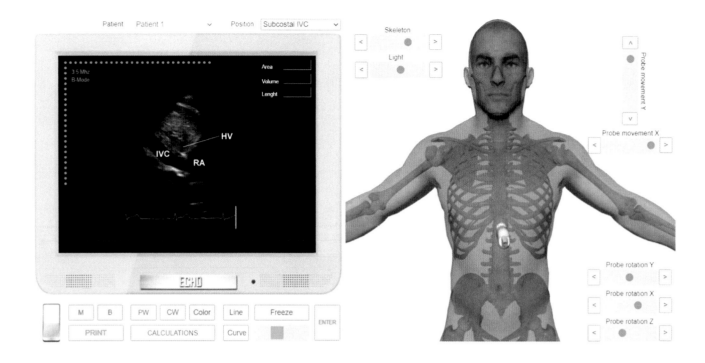

Subcostal View

SUBCOSTAL VIEW OF THE INFERIOR VENA CAVA

This approach makes it possible to study Inferior Vena Cava and Hepatic Veins. The study of the inferior Vena cava and its collaboration with the phases of respiration is mandatory in all patients. It is used for assessing Pressure in the Pulmonary Artery (typically, the diameter of the inferior Vena cava decreases by 50% during inspiration).

First, we must find Subcostal 4 Chamber View to obtain this position. After Turning the transducer (See Operations on Transducer) 90 degrees counterclockwise. Transducer Marker is oriented toward the patient's face (12 o'clock).

The following heart structures are visualized on the screen:

- **IVC** - Inferior Vena Cava.
- **HV** - Hepatic Vein.
- **RA** - Right Atrium.

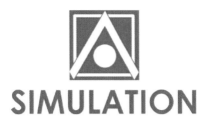

SIMULATION

Subcostal View of the Inferior Vena Cava

Echocardiography Online Simulator
MyEchocardiography.com

- Go to the link https://simulation.myechocardiography.com/

- Run Echocardiography Online Simulator using the **On/Off** Button

- Choose the patient from the list **<<Patient>>** Patient   Patient 1   ⌄

- Switch Echocardiography Simulator to **B-Mode**   B   * Initially Simulator is set to B-Mode.

- Using Slider and Buttons **<<Skeleton>>**   < ● >   Choose appropriate transparency level.

- Choose position " **Subcostal IVC**" from the List **<<Positions>>**   Position   Subcostal IVC   ⌄
  or Find the position with the 3D Transducer.

- To change the patient, click the **On/Off** Button

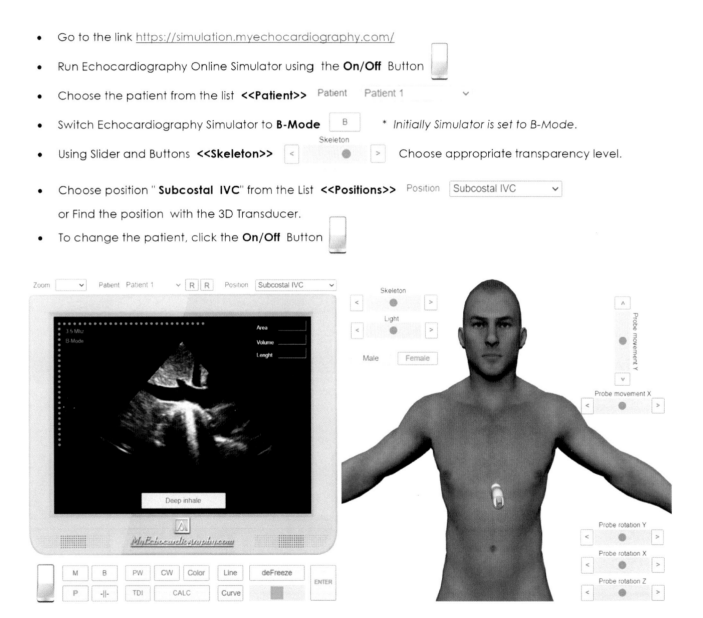

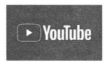

https://youtu.be/SAeNKsSQFhE

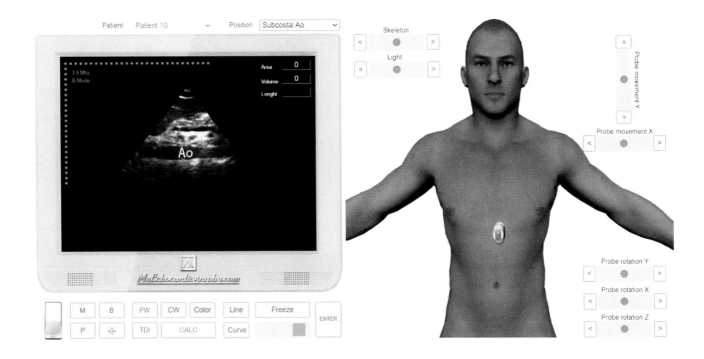

Subcostal View

SUBCOSTAL VIEW OF THE AORTA

This approach is used to study the Abdominal Aorta (long axis)

From the subcostal view of the IVC, the subcostal view of the abdominal aorta is obtained by angling the sound beam to the patient's left side (left lateral).

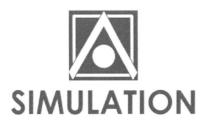

SIMULATION

Subcostal View of the Aorta

Echocardiography Online Simulator

MyEchocardiography.com

- Go to the link https://simulation.myechocardiography.com/

- Run Echocardiography Online Simulator using the **On/Off** Button

- Choose the patient from the list **<<Patient>>** Patient   Patient 1 ⌄

- Switch Echocardiography Simulator to **B-Mode**   B   * Initially Simulator is set to B-Mode.

- Using Slider and Buttons **<<Skeleton>>**   <   ●   >   Choose appropriate transparency level.

- Choose position " **Subcostal Ao**" from the List **<<Positions>>**   Position   Subcostal Ao ⌄

  or Find the position with the 3D Transducer.

- To change the patient, click the **On/Off** Button

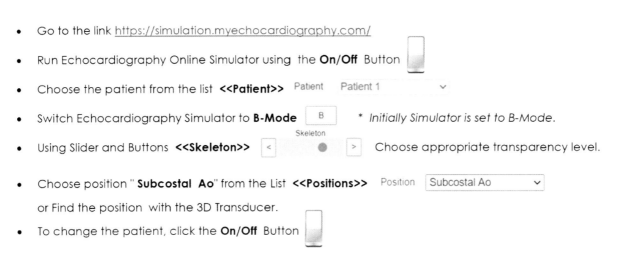

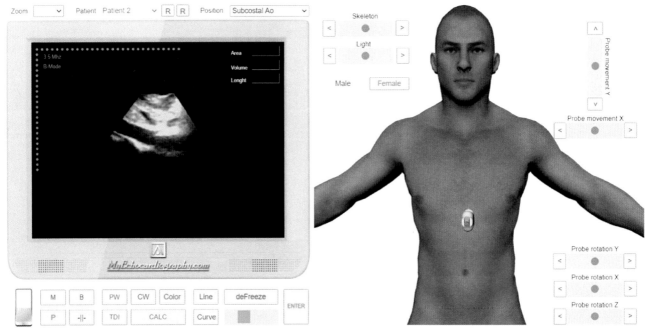

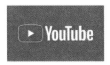

https://youtu.be/JXMP_4pxoGU

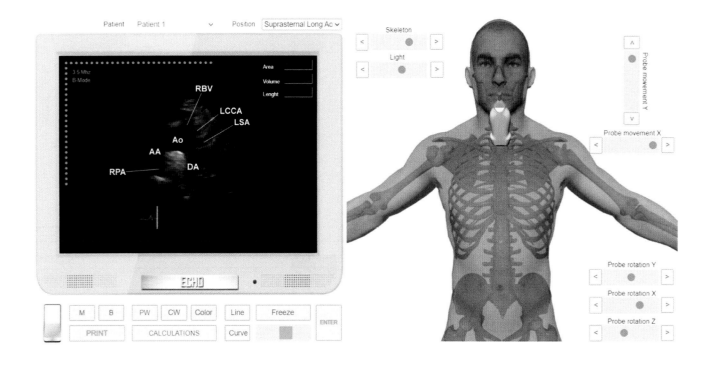

Suprasternal View

SUPRASTERNAL VIEW. LONG AXIS OF AORTIC ARCH

The suprasternal approach makes it possible to study the aortic arch, the right branch of the pulmonary artery, and often the superior Vena cava. It is used to study the flow in these vessels. The patient is lying on his back with his head turned 45 degrees.

The Transducer will interfere with the jugular fossa. The Transducer Marker should be pointing up. The Central ultrasound beam is directed downward to obtain the maximum diameter of the aortic arch along its entire length.

The following heart structures are visualized on the screen:

- **AA** - Ascending Aorta.
- **Ao** - Aortic Arch.
- **DA** - Descending Aorta.
- **RPA** - Right Pulmonary Artery.
- **RBV** - Left Brachiocephalic Vein.
- **LCCA** - Left Common Carotid Artery.
- **LSA** - Left Subclavian Artery.

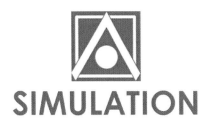

SIMULATION
Suprasternal View, the Long Axis of Aortic Arch

Echocardiography Online Simulator
MyEchocardiography.com

- Go to the link https://simulation.myechocardiography.com/

- Run Echocardiography Online Simulator using the **On/Off** Button

- Choose the patient from the list **<<Patient>>**   Patient   Patient 1 ⌄

- Switch Echocardiography Simulator to **B-Mode**   B   * Initially Simulator is set to B-Mode.

- Using Slider and Buttons **<<Skeleton>>**   < ● >   Choose appropriate transparency level.

- Choose position " **Suprasternal Long Ao** " from the List **<<Positions>>**   Position   Suprasternal Long Ao ⌄
  or Find the position with the 3D Transducer.

- To change the patient, click the **On/Off** Button

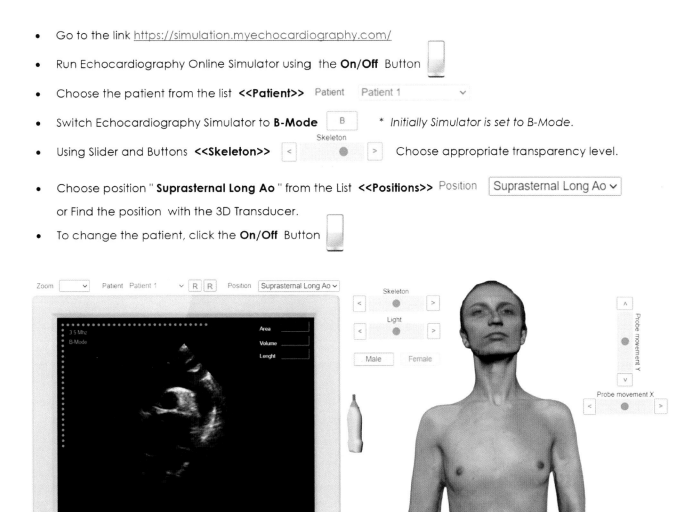

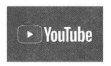

https://youtu.be/O843zjz08LQ

ONE-DIMENSIONAL ECHOCARDIOGRAPHY

M-Mode

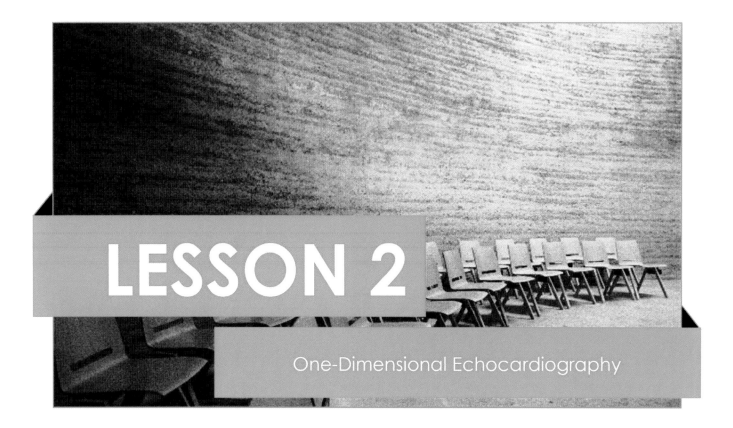

LESSON 2

One-Dimensional Echocardiography

The one-dimensional examination is mainly carried out from the parasternal position along the long axis of the heart. The angle of inclination of the m-modal cursor is chosen so that the ultrasound beam crosses the mitral valve, aortic valve, and left ventricle.

Nowadays, one-dimensional echocardiography is mainly used as an additional measurement method. The cursor should be positioned strictly perpendicular to the structures of the heart. In this case, measurements can be made with great accuracy.

The distinct advantage of M-modal echocardiography is its high resolution. Therefore, one-dimensional echocardiogram provides essential information from rapidly moving structures. For example, a vibration of the anterior mitral leaflet cannot be detected on a 2D echocardiogram.

The advantage of two-dimensional echocardiography is its two-dimensional nature. On the other hand, one-dimensional echocardiography does not provide spatial information.

On the M-modal graph, distances are located vertically, time is horizontal. The graph gives the following information:

- **Time** - on the horizontal axis.
- **Distance** - on the vertical axis.
- **Saturation (density)** of the ultrasound signal - on the display the structure with different brightness (echogenicity).

One-dimensional (M-Mode) Examinations:

- M-modal examination of the mitral valve.
- M-modal examination of the aorta and aortic valve.
- M-modal examination of the left ventricle.

User can Simulate all the basic M-Mode examinations by Echocardiography Online Simulator MyEchocardiography.com

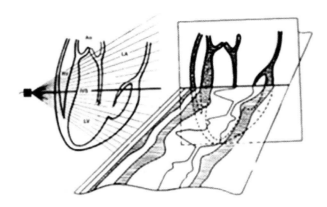

The relationship between one-dimensional and two-dimensional echocardiography.

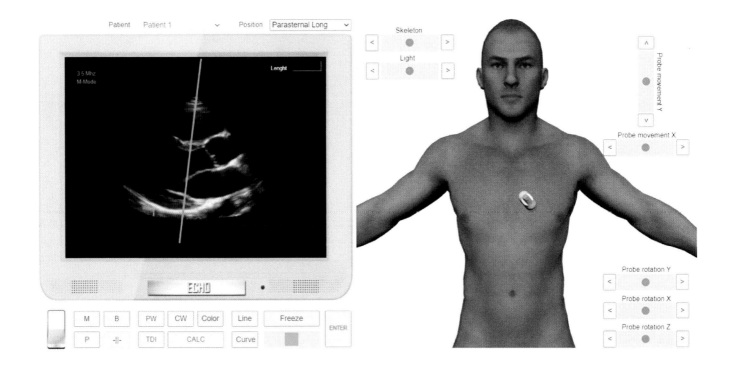

M-Mode

ONE-DIMENSIONAL EXAMINATION OF THE MITRAL VALVE

For the One-dimensional study of the Mitral valve better to use a parasternal approach (the long axis of the heart). The M-modal cursor should be perpendicular to the long axis of the heart and cross the ends of the mitral valve leaflets.

On the display, from top to bottom, we see the following structures:

- **AWRV** - Anterior wall of the right ventricle.
- **RV** - Right ventricular cavity.
- **IVS** - Interventricular septum.
- **LV** - Left ventricular cavity.
- **ALMV** - Anterior leaflet of the mitral valve.
- **PLMV** - Posterior leaflet of the mitral valve.
- **PWLV** - Posterior wall of the left ventricle.
- **PE** - Parietal pericardium.

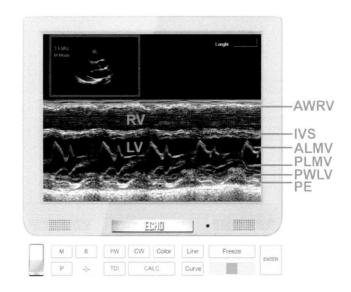

One-Dimensional Echocardiography

This position makes it possible to study the structure of the mitral valve and the nature of its movement.

In the typical case, there is an M-shaped movement of the anterior leaflet and a W-shaped movement of the posterior leaflet of the mitral valve.

On the curve of the movement of the anterior leaflet, the following sections are distinguished:

- **C-D** interval - Left ventricular systole and leaflet closure.
- **D-E** interval - Rapid filling phase and opening of the leaflets.
- **E-F** interval - Incomplete closing of the leaflets in the slow filling phase.
- **A wave** - Secondary divergence of the leaflets in left atrial systole.

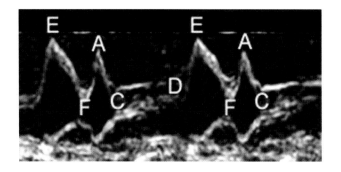

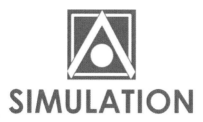

SIMULATION

M-MODAL EXAMINATION OF THE MITRAL VALVE

Echocardiography Online Simulator
MyEchocardiography.com

- Go to the link https://simulation.myechocardiography.com/

- Run Echocardiography Online Simulator using the **On/Off** Button

- Choose the patient from the list **<<Patient>>** Patient   Patient 1   ∨

- Switch Echocardiography Simulator to **M-Mode**   M   * Initially Simulator is set to B-Mode.

- Choose position " **Parasternal Long** " from the List **<<Positions>>**   Position   Parasternal Long   ∨
  or Find the position with the 3D Transducer.

- Cross the ends of the Mitral Valve leaflets with the M-modal cursor and click.

- To change the patient, click the **On/Off** Button

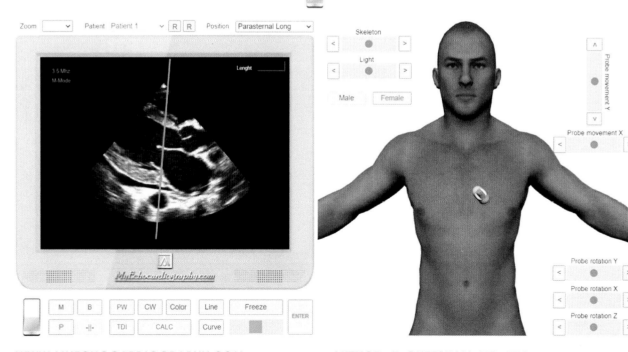

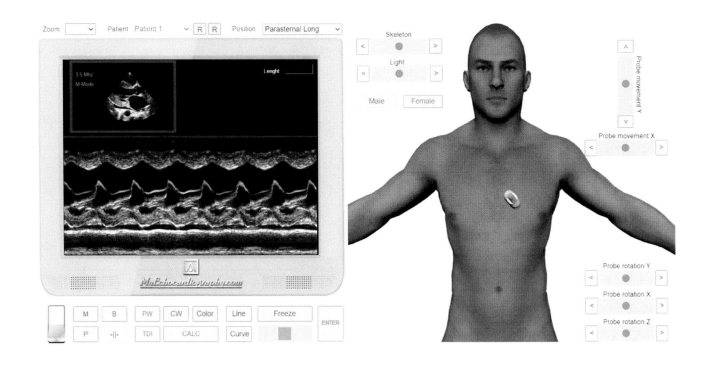

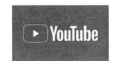

https://youtu.be/FzYc6aCVCYU

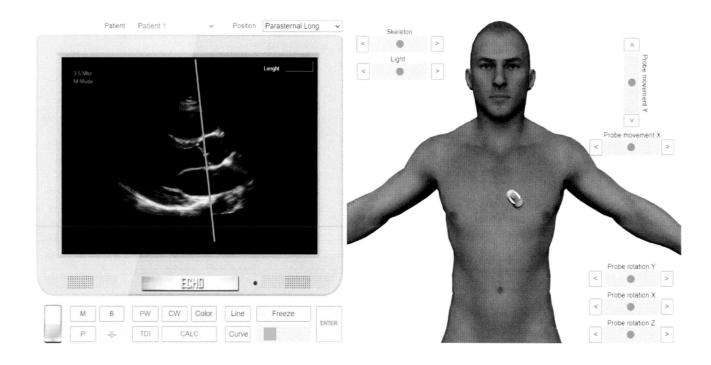

M-Mode

ONE-DIMENSIONAL EXAMINATION OF THE AORTA AND AORTIC VALVE

For the One-dimensional study of the Aorta and Aortic valve better to use a parasternal approach (the long axis of the heart). The M-modal cursor should cross the Aortic valve.

On the display, from top to bottom, we see the following structures:

AWRV - Anterior wall of the right ventricle.
RV - Right ventricular cavity.
AWA - Anterior wall of the Aorta..
RCC - Right coronary cusp of Aortic Valve.
NCC - Non-coronary cusp of Aortic Valve.
PWA - Posterior wall of the Aorta.
LA - Left Atrial cavity.

PWLA - Posterior wall of the left Atrium.
Only two aortic valve cusps can be examined in one-dimensional echocardiography: the right coronary cusp and the non-coronary cusp. They diverge with the left ventricular systole, join with the diastole and create a curve that resembles a rectangle.

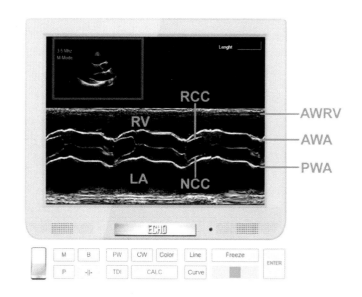

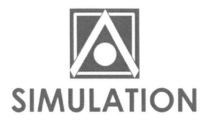

SIMULATION
M-MODAL EXAMINATION OF THE AORTA
AND AORTIC VALVE

Echocardiography Online Simulator
MyEchocardiography.com

- Go to the link https://simulation.myechocardiography.com/

- Run Echocardiography Online Simulator using the **On/Off** Button

- Choose the patient from the list **<<Patient>>** Patient   Patient 1   ⌄

- Switch Echocardiography Simulator to **M-Mode**   M   * Initially Simulator is set to B-Mode.

- Choose position "**Parasternal Long**" from the List **<<Positions>>** Position Parasternal Long ⌄
  or Find the position with the 3D Transducer.

- Cross the ends of the Aortic Valve leaflets with the M-modal cursor and click.

- To change the patient, click the **On/Off** Button

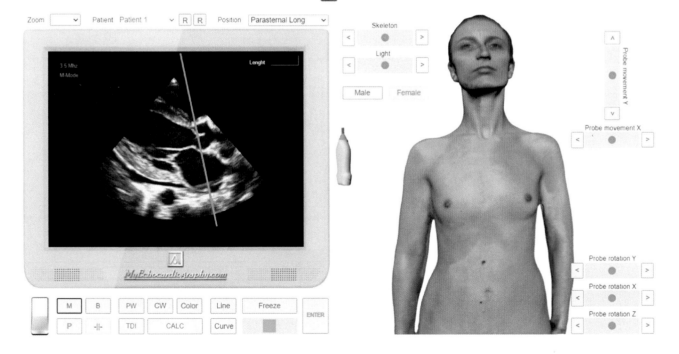

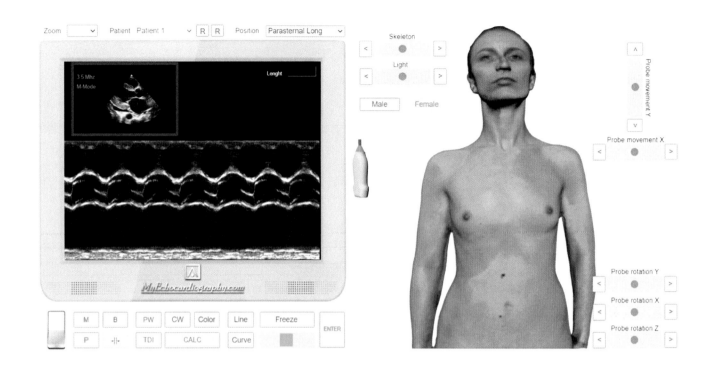

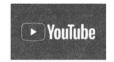

https://youtu.be/7EPoAA2fyCQ

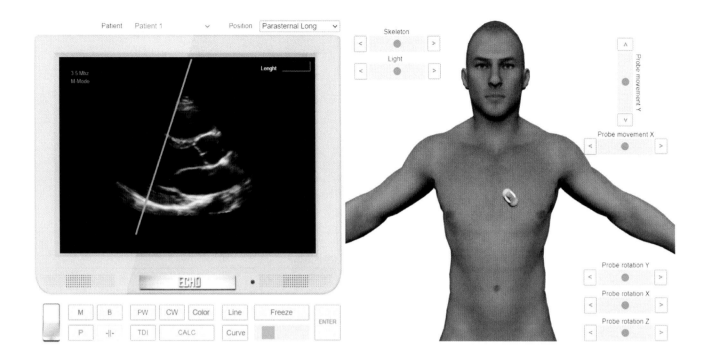

M-Mode

ONE-DIMENSIONAL EXAMINATION OF THE LEFT VENTRICLE

For the One-dimensional study of the Left Ventricle better to use a parasternal approach (the long axis of the heart). The M-modal cursor should be perpendicular to the long axis of the heart and cross the Left Ventricle at the level of papillary muscles.

On the display, from top to bottom, we see the following structures:

- **AWRV** - Anterior wall of the right ventricle.
- **RV** - Right ventricular cavity.
- **IVS** - Interventricular septum.
- **LV** - Left ventricular cavity.
- **PWLV** - Posterior wall of the left ventricle.
- **PE** - Pericardium.

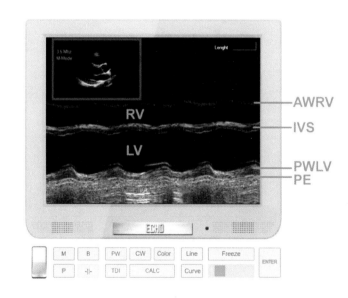

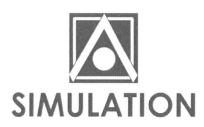

SIMULATION
M-MODAL EXAMINATION OF THE LEFT VENTRICLE

Echocardiography Online Simulator
MyEchocardiography.com

- Go to the link https://simulation.myechocardiography.com/

- Run Echocardiography Online Simulator using the **On/Off** Button

- Choose the patient from the list **<<Patient>>** Patient   Patient 1 ⌄

- Switch Echocardiography Simulator to **M-Mode**   M   * Initially Simulator is set to B-Mode.

- Choose position " **Parasternal Long** " from the List **<<Positions>>** Position Parasternal Long ⌄
  or Find the position with the 3D Transducer.

- Cross the Left Ventricle with the M-modal cursor and click.

- To change the patient, click the **On/Off** Button

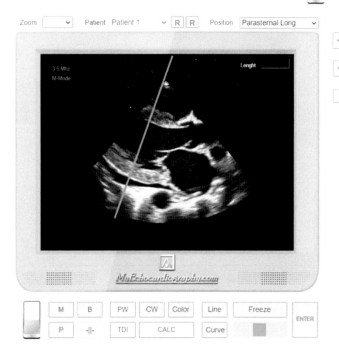

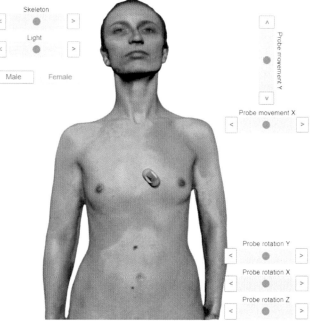

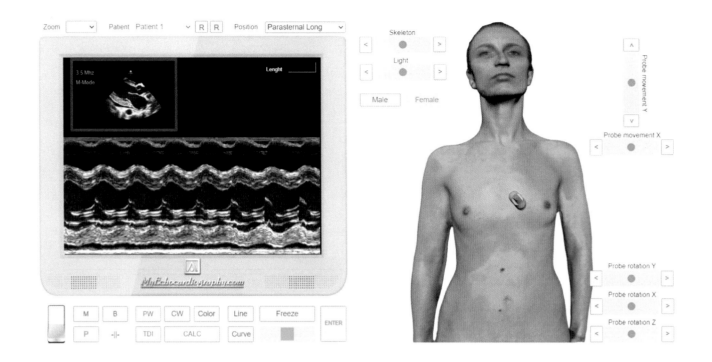

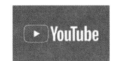

https://youtu.be/O_tLjSGTaJ4

SPECTRAL DOPPLER

PW and CW Doppler

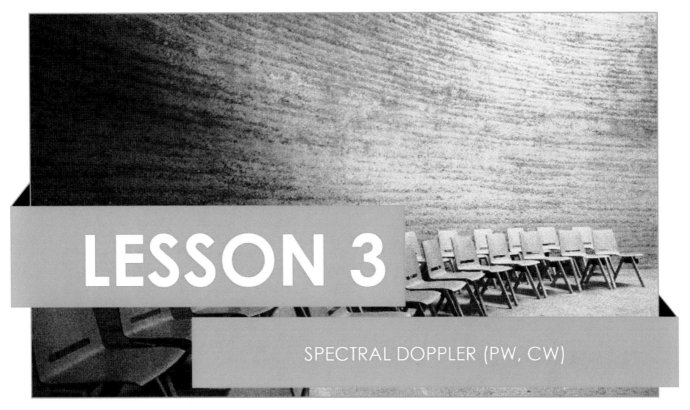

LESSON 3

SPECTRAL DOPPLER (PW, CW)

Spectral Doppler Information:

- Flow velocity.
- Flow direction.
- Signal time.
- Signal intensity.

The flow velocity is plotted on the y-axis. When there is no flow, only the baseline is visible on the display.

The direction of flow is also shown on the y-axis. Flows directed towards the transducer are located on top of the baseline, flows that are directed away from the transducer are located at the bottom of the baseline.

The Signal intensity is shown as the brightness of the stream. A brighter Spectrum corresponds to higher intensity (many red cells are moving in this area) and vice versa.

The signal Time is plotted on the x-axis.

When examined from a Pulsed Wave Doppler (PW), the same piezoelectric element sends and receives a signal. With a continuous wave Doppler (CW), one piezoelectric element sends a signal, and the other acts as a receiver.

LESSON CONTENT

Spectral Doppler. PW and CW Doppler examinations:

- Transmitral diastolic flow Spectral Doppler
- Trans Tricuspid diastolic flow Spectral Doppler
- Pulmonary vein flow Spectral Doppler
- Left ventricular outflow tract (LVOT) flow Spectral Doppler
- Ascending aortic flow Spectral Doppler
- Right ventricular outflow tract (RVOT) flow Spectral Doppler
- Pulmonary artery flow Spectral Doppler
- Inferior vena cava (IVC) flow Spectral Doppler
- Descending aortic flow Spectral Doppler

SPECTRAL DOPPLER

The place where the signal is analyzed is called the

Sample Volume.

The Sample volume will appear on the screen when switching to the PW or CW mode. It can be moved to any position where we want to study the characteristics of the flow.

The point where the Sample volume is located is called the **Baseline**.

The superiority of PW over CW is the depth resolution that CW does not have. In PW mode, studying the flow characteristics *at the Sample Volume point* at different depths is possible.

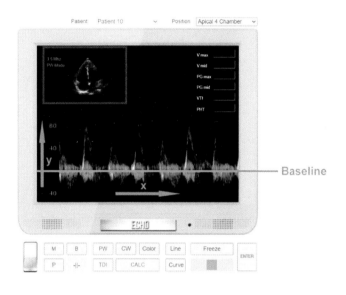

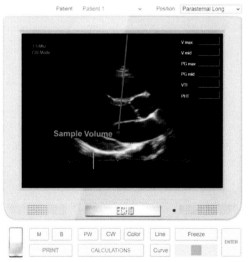

Nyquist limit

The main disadvantage of pulse wave (PW) Doppler versus continuous wave (CW) is the existence of the Nyquist limit. The maximum speed that can be learned in PW mode is called the Nyquist limit. If velocity is higher than this limit spectrum will be distorted.

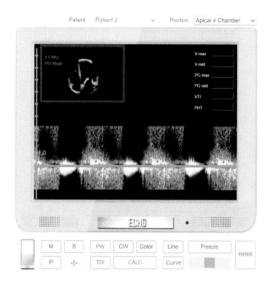

PW doppler examination. Velocity is higher than Nyquist limit and spectrum is distorted

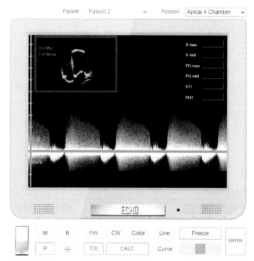

The same flow by CW Doppler

In CW mode, it is possible to examine the flow at any speed. The main disadvantage of CW Doppler is that it has no depth resolution.

Nyquist limit = PRF/2

PRF - Pulse repetition frequency

Spectral Doppler (PW, CW) Examinations

- Transmitral diastolic flow Spectral Doppler
- Trans Tricuspid diastolic flow Spectral Doppler
- Pulmonary vein flow Spectral Doppler
- Left ventricular outflow tract (LVOT) flow Spectral Doppler
- Ascending aortic flow Spectral Doppler
- Right ventricular outflow tract (RVOT) flow Spectral Doppler
- Pulmonary artery flow Spectral Doppler
- Inferior vena cava (IVC) flow Spectral Doppler
- Descending aortic flow Spectral Doppler

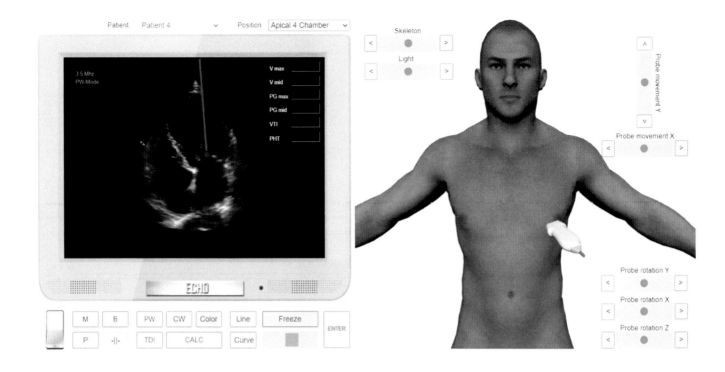

SPECTRAL DOPPLER (PW, CW)

TRANS-MITRAL DIASTOLIC FLOW

The apical four-chamber view is the best position to study trans-mitral diastolic flow by spectral Doppler (PW, CW). In this case, the flow is more parallel to the ultrasonic beam. The control volume is placed at the level of the end of the open leaflets of the mitral valve.

Normal trans-mitral flow occurs only in the diastole phase.
The flow is towards the transducer, is recorded from the top of the baseline, and is biphasic.

- **E** - Early diastolic filling.
- **A** - Atrial contraction.

Diastole can be divided into two more phases:

- **IVRT** - Isovolumetric relaxation time. It can be measured if simultaneously studying the transmitral diastolic flow and the flow in the outflow tract of the left ventricle. In this case, the sample volume is placed at the border of these two streams.

- **L** - Diastasis, a small wave between E and A, is more common in children and adolescents.

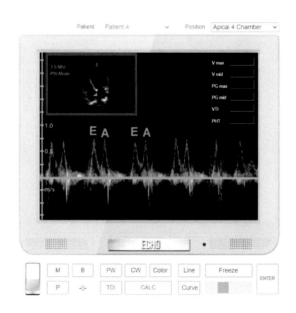

Using the trans-mitral diastolic flow spectrogram the following parameters can be measured and calculated:

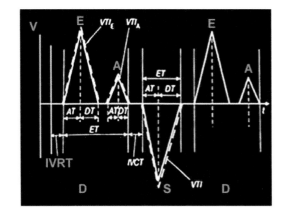

- **AT** (Acceleration Time) - The time from the opening of the mitral valve to the peak flow.
- **DT** (Deceleration Time) - the time from the Peak to Baseline.
- **ET** (Ejection Time) - The time from opening to closing the mitral valve.
- **Vmid** (Average Flow Velocity) - The sum of the flow velocities measured every 2 seconds, divided by the number of measurements.
- **VTI** (Velocity Time Integral) - *VTI = Vmid x ET*
- **Vmax** - Maximum flow velocity.
- **IVRT** - Isovolumetric relaxation time.
- **IVST** - Isovolumetric contraction time.

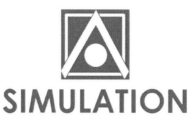

SIMULATION
TRANS-MITRAL DIASTOLIC FLOW PW AND CW Doppler

Echocardiography Online Simulator
MyEchocardiography.com

- Go to the link https://simulation.myechocardiography.com/

- Run Echocardiography Online Simulator using the **On/Off** Button

- Choose the patient from the list **<<Patient>>**   Patient   [Patient 1   ∨]

- Switch Echocardiography Simulator to **B-Mode** [B]   * *Initially Simulator is set to B-Mode.*

- Choose position " **Apical 4 Chamber**" from the List **<<Positions>>**   Position [Apical 4 Chamber ∨]
  or Find the position with the 3D Transducer.

- Click the button **<<PW>>** to move to Pulse Wave Spectral Doppler (PW) or **<<CW>>** to move to Continuous Wave Spectral Doppler (CW)

- Place **Sample Volume** at the level of the end of the open leaflets of the mitral valve and **click.**

- To change the patient, click the **On/Off** Button

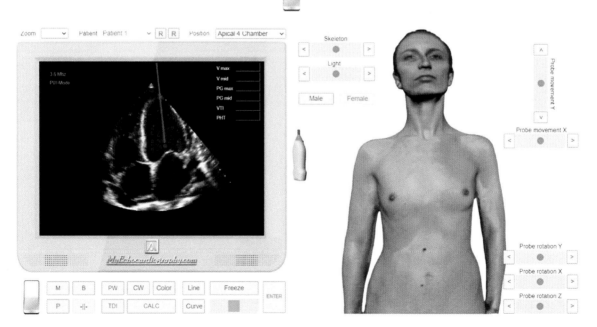

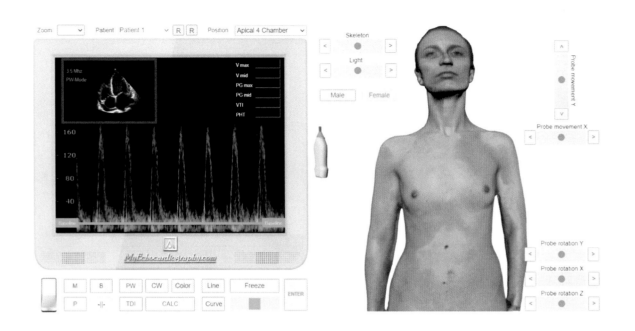

https://youtu.be/amNi3nygca4

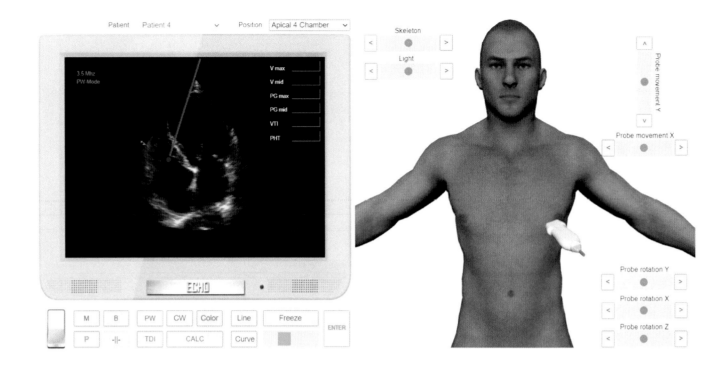

SPECTRAL DOPPLER (PW, CW)

TRANS-TRICUSPID DIASTOLIC FLOW

The apical four-chamber view is the best position to study trans-tricuspid diastolic flow by spectral Doppler (PW, CW). In this case, the flow is more parallel to the ultrasonic beam. The control volume is placed at the level of the end of the open leaflets of the tricuspid valve.

Normal trans-mitral flow occurs only in the diastole phase. In 50-65% of cases, physiological regurgitation is observed on the tricuspid valve.
The flow is towards the transducer, is recorded from the top of the baseline, and is biphasic.

- **E** - Early diastolic filling.
- **A** - Atrial contraction.

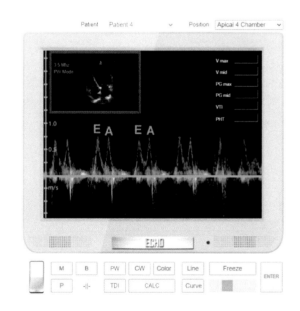

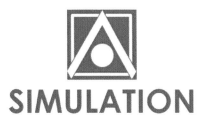

SIMULATION
TRANS-TRICUSPID DIASTOLIC FLOW PW AND CW Doppler

Echocardiography Online Simulator
MyEchocardiography.com

- Go to the link https://simulation.myechocardiography.com/

- Run Echocardiography Online Simulator using the **On/Off** Button

- Choose the patient from the list **<<Patient>>** Patient [Patient 1 ⌄]

- Switch Echocardiography Simulator to **B-Mode** [B]   *Initially Simulator is set to B-Mode.*

- Choose position " **Apical 4 Chamber**" from the List **<<Positions>>** Position [Apical 4 Chamber ⌄]
  or Find the position with the 3D Transducer.

- Click the button **<<PW>>** to move to Pulse Wave Spectral Doppler (PW) or **<<CW>>** to move to Continuous Wave Spectral Doppler (CW)

- Place **Sample Volume** at the level of the end of the open leaflets of the tricuspid valve and **click.**

- To change the patient, click the **On/Off** Button

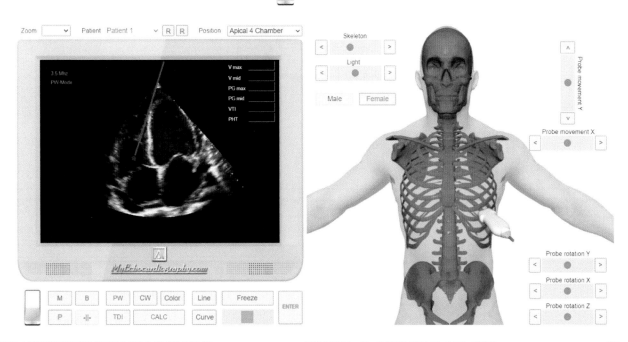

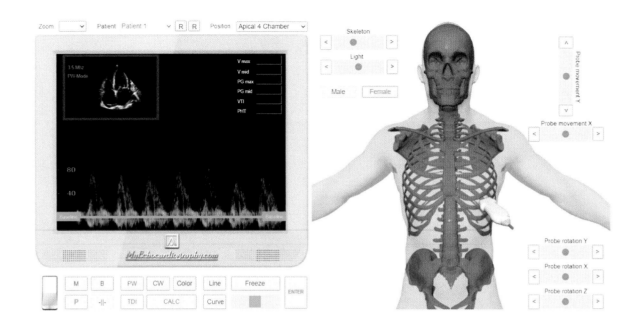

https://youtu.be/k4109iSMuyo

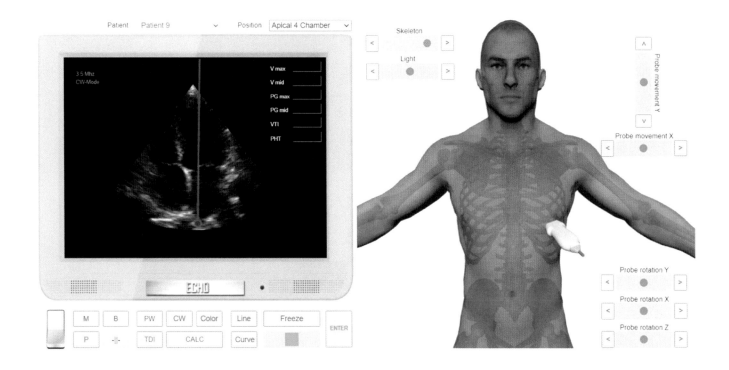

SPECTRAL DOPPLER (PW, CW)

PULMONARY VEINS FLOW

The apical four-chamber view is the best position to study Pulmonary Veins flow by spectral Doppler (PW, CW). The control volume is placed in the Pulmonary Veins at 10-20 mm depth.

Normally, the flow is observed both in the systole and diastole phases. Consists of Systolic, Diastolic, and Atrial components.
The speed of the systolic phase is greater than the diastolic. Therefore, they register on top of the baseline. With the contraction of the left atrium, a small reversion of blood is observed, which is reported below the baseline.

- **S** - Systolic phase.
- **D** - Diastolic phase.
- **Ar** - Atrial Component

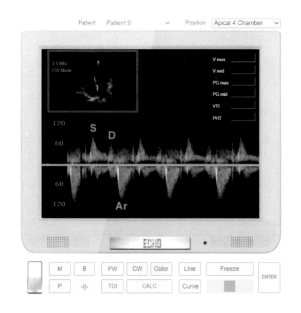

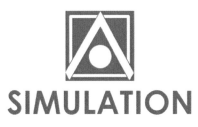

SIMULATION

PULMONARY VEINS FLOW PW AND CW
Doppler

Echocardiography Online Simulator
MyEchocardiography.com

- Go to the link https://simulation.myechocardiography.com/

- Run Echocardiography Online Simulator using the **On/Off** Button

- Choose the patient from the list **<<Patient>>** Patient   Patient 1 ⌄

- Switch Echocardiography Simulator to **B-Mode** [B]   * *Initially Simulator is set to B-Mode.*

- Choose position " **Apical 4 Chamber**" from the List **<<Positions>>** Position   Apical 4 Chamber ⌄
  or Find the position with the 3D Transducer.

- Click the button **<<PW>>** to move to Pulse Wave Spectral Doppler (PW) or **<<CW>>** to move to Continuous Wave Spectral Doppler (CW)

- Place **Sample Volume** in the Pulmonary vein and **click.**

- To change the patient, click the **On/Off** Button

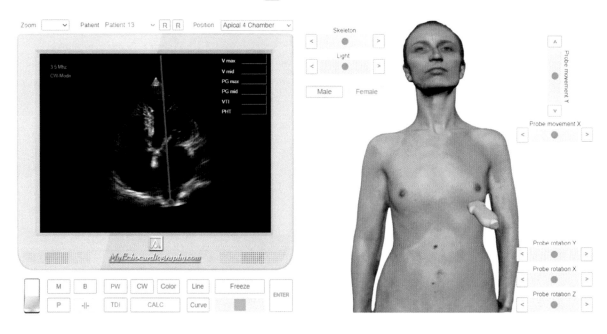

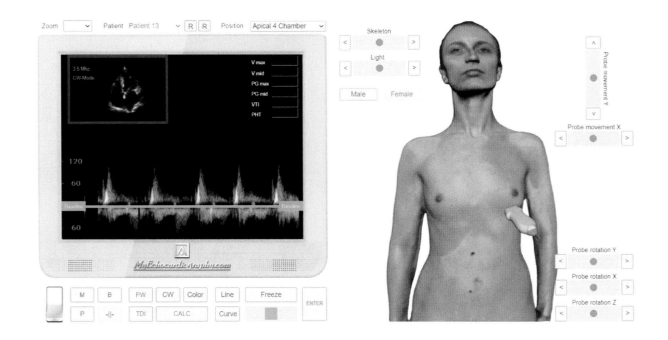

https://youtu.be/T0nlo2XwDrE

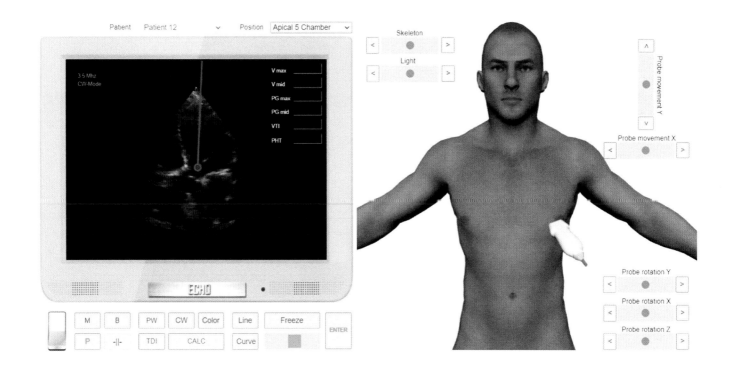

SPECTRAL DOPPLER (PW, CW)

LEFT VENTRICULAR OUTFLOW TRACT (LVOT) FLOW SPECTRAL DOPPLER

The apical five-chamber position is the best choice for studying left ventricular outflow tract flow. In this position, the flow is almost parallel to the ultrasonic beam. It is also possible to use the left parasternal approach, the long axis of the heart.

The Sample Volume is proximal to the aortic valve (5-10 mm from the valve, towards the left ventricle). The flow will almost always exceed the Nyquist limit; therefore, a continuous wave Doppler is better for examination.

Typically, the flow in the outflow tract of the left ventricle occurs in the systole phase and is directed toward the aorta. The flow is directed away from the transducer and located below the baseline.

In the aorta, the flow speed is slightly higher than in the outflow tract of the left ventricle. Therefore, if there is no aortic stenosis, we can limit ourselves only to studying the outflow tract flow (In this case, the flow in the aorta is almost the same as in the LV outflow tract).

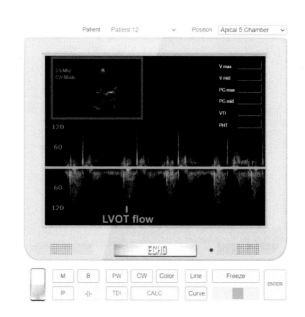

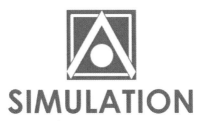

SIMULATION
LEFT VENTRICULAR OUTFLOW TRACT (LVOT) FLOW PW AND CW DOPPLER

Echocardiography Online Simulator
MyEchocardiography.com

- Go to the link https://simulation.myechocardiography.com/

- Run Echocardiography Online Simulator using the **On/Off** Button

- Choose the patient from the list **<<Patient>>** Patient [Patient 1 ⌄]

- Switch Echocardiography Simulator to **B-Mode** [B] * Initially Simulator is set to B-Mode.

- Choose position " **Apical 5 Chamber**" from the List **<<Positions>>** Position [Apical 5 Chamber ⌄] or Find the position with the 3D Transducer.

- Click the button **<<PW>>** to move to Pulse Wave Spectral Doppler (PW) or **<<CW>>** to move to Continuous Wave Spectral Doppler (CW)

- Place **Sample Volume** proximal to the aortic valve (at a distance of 5-10 mm from the valve, toward the left ventricle) and click.

- To change the patient, click the **On/Off** Button

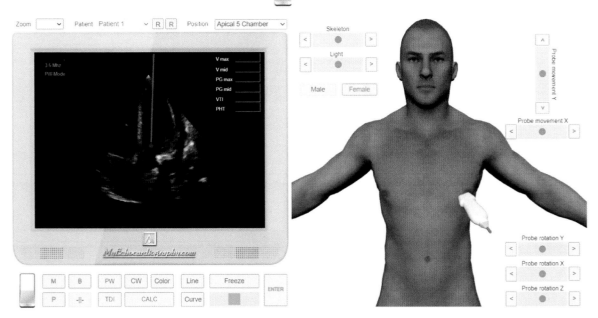

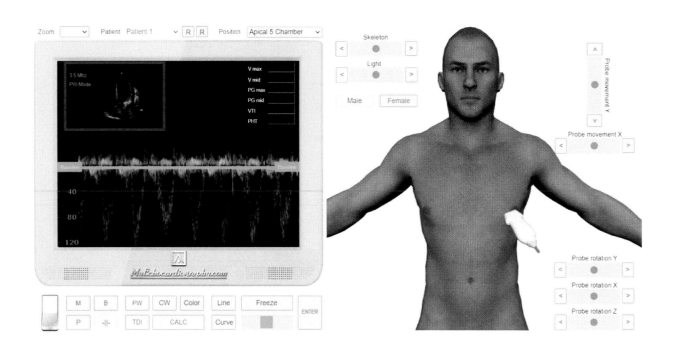

https://youtu.be/nAJ-ys1UpZU

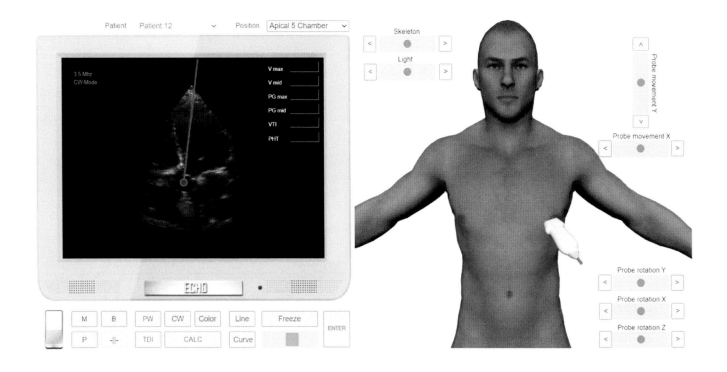

SPECTRAL DOPPLER (PW, CW)
ASCENDING AORTIC FLOW SPECTRAL DOPPLER

The Apical Five Chamber position is the best choice for studying Ascending aortic flow. In this position, the flow is almost parallel to the ultrasonic beam. It is also possible to use the left parasternal approach, the long axis of the heart, and the Suprasternal Approach.

The Sample Volume is placed on top of the aortic valve cusps. The flow will almost always exceed the Nyquist limit; therefore, a continuous wave Doppler is better to use for examination.

Typically, the flow in the outflow tract of the left ventricle occurs in the systole phase and is directed toward the aorta. The flow is directed away from the transducer and located below the baseline.
In the aorta, the flow speed is slightly higher than in the outflow tract of the left ventricle. Therefore, if there is no aortic stenosis, we can limit ourselves only to studying the outflow tract flow (In this case, the flow in the aorta is almost the same as in the LV outflow tract).

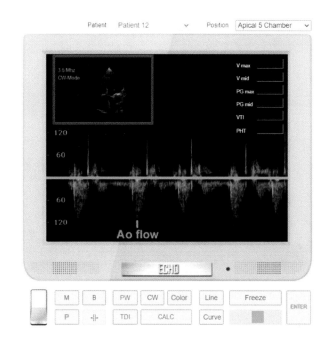

In the case of the Suprasternal Approach, The flow is directed towards the transducer and located above the baseline.

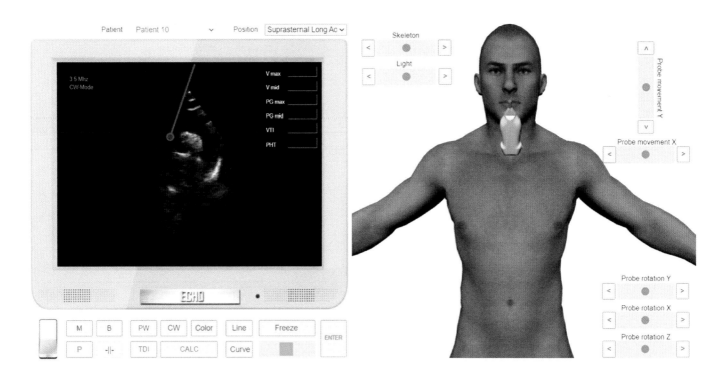

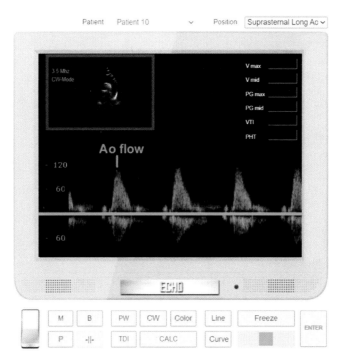

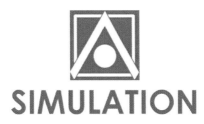

SIMULATION
ASCENDING AORTIC FLOW PW AND CW DOPPLER

Echocardiography Online Simulator
MyEchocardiography.com

- Go to the link https://simulation.myechocardiography.com/

- Run Echocardiography Online Simulator using the **On/Off** Button

- Choose the patient from the list **<<Patient>>** Patient [Patient 1 ∨]

- Switch Echocardiography Simulator to **B-Mode** [B]   * *Initially Simulator is set to B-Mode.*

- Choose position " **Apical 5 Chamber**" or **"Suprasternal Long"** or **"Parasternal Long"**

  from the List **<<Positions>>** Position [Apical 5 Chamber ∨] or Find the position with the 3D Transducer.

- Click the button **<<PW>>** to move to Pulse Wave Spectral Doppler (PW) or **<<CW>>** to move to Continuous Wave Spectral Doppler (CW)

- Place **Sample Volume** on the top of the aortic valve cusps and click.

- To change the patient, click the **On/Off** Button

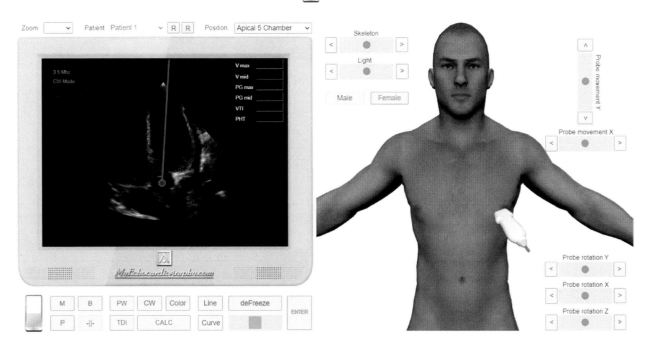

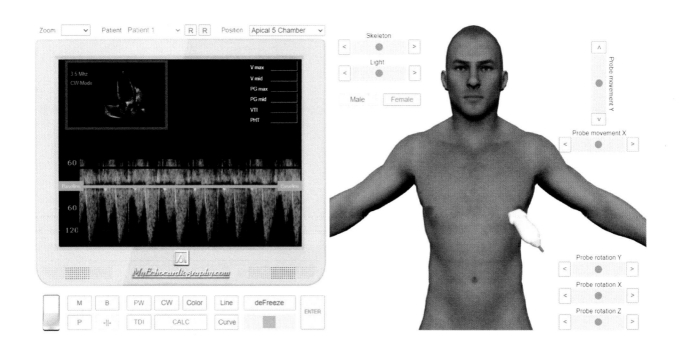

https://youtu.be/xgKSMdP7f7I

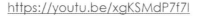

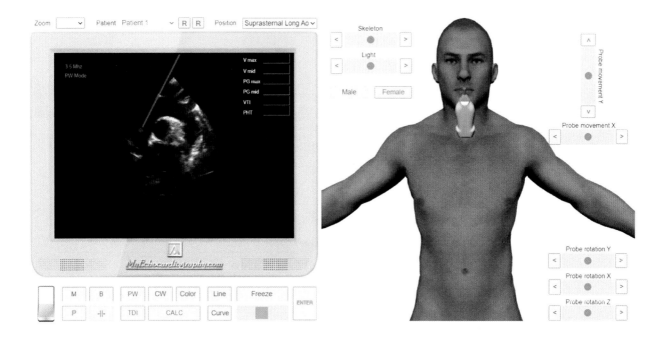

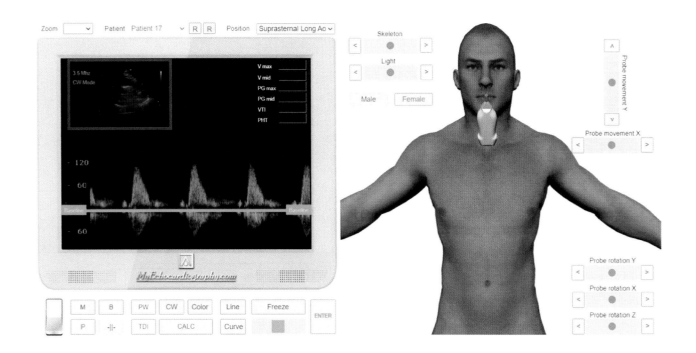

https://youtu.be/rvJWt-u7wCc

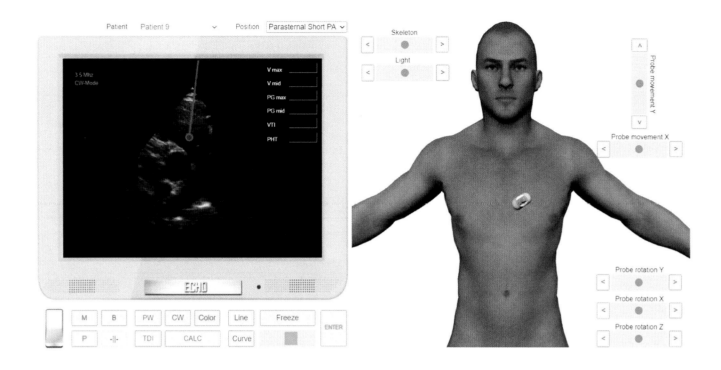

SPECTRAL DOPPLER (PW, CW)

RIGHT VENTRICULAR OUTFLOW TRACT (RVOT) FLOW

The study is better performed from a Parasternal Approach, the short axis of the heart, at the level of the Aortic Valve or Pulmonary Artery.

The Sample Volume is placed under the cusps of the pulmonary valve, towards the right ventricle (1 cm proximally).

Flow occurs in the diastole phase and is directed from the right ventricle to the pulmonary artery, away from the transducer, and below the Baseline. The flow, in contrast to the aortic, has a small amplitude.

In 50-65% of cases, physiological regurgitation is observed on the pulmonary valve.

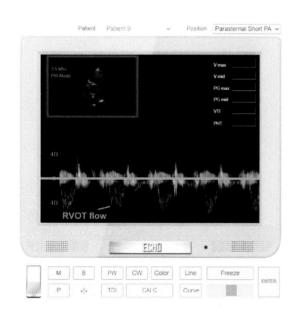

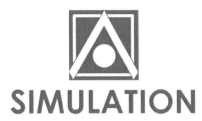

SIMULATION

RIGHT VENTRICULAR OUTFLOW TRACT (RVOT) FLOW PW AND CW Doppler

Echocardiography Online Simulator
MyEchocardiography.com

- Go to the link https://simulation.myechocardiography.com/

- Run Echocardiography Online Simulator using the **On/Off** Button

- Choose the patient from the list **<<Patient>>** Patient | Patient 1 ∨ |

- Switch Echocardiography Simulator to **B-Mode** | B | * Initially Simulator is set to B-Mode.

- Choose position " **"Parasternal Short PA"** or **"Parasternal Short Ao "** From the list **<<Positions>>**
  or Find the position with the 3D Transducer.

- Click the button **<<PW>>** to move to Pulse Wave Spectral Doppler (PW) or **<<CW>>** to move to Continuous Wave Spectral Doppler (CW)

- Place **Sample Volume** above the Pulmonary artery valve and **click.**

- To change the patient, click the **On/Off** Button

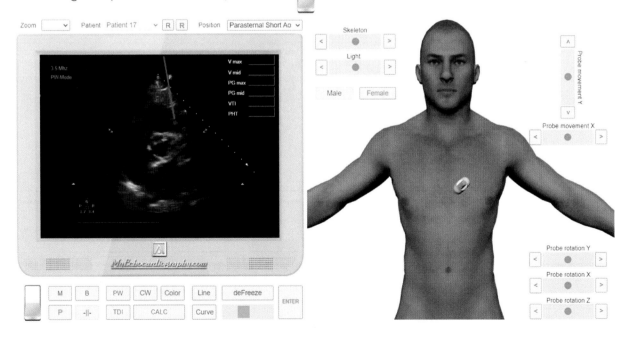

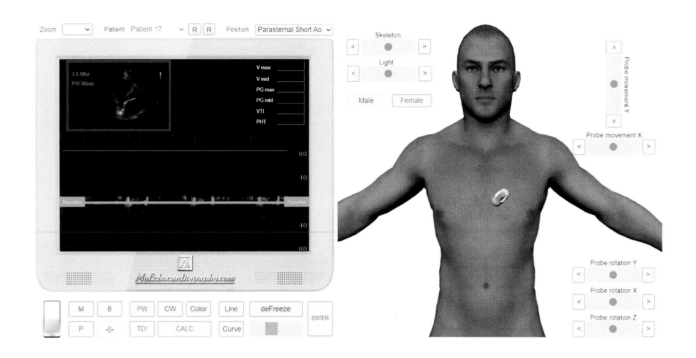

https://youtu.be/4_VMTVmAEC4

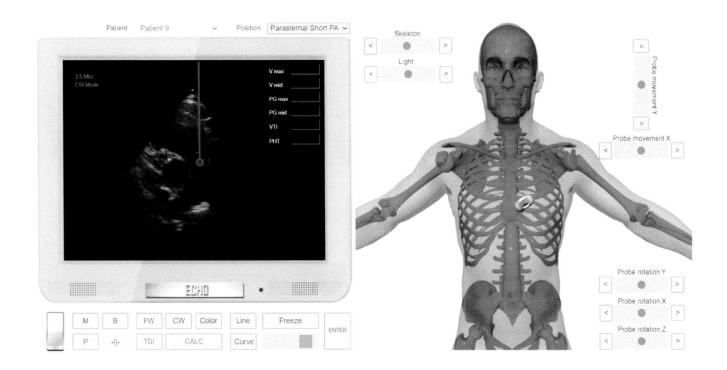

SPECTRAL DOPPLER (PW, CW)

PULMONARY ARTERY FLOW SPECTRAL DOPPLER

The study is better performed from a Parasternal Approach, the heart's short axis, at the Pulmonary Artery level. Therefore, the Sample Volume is placed in the Pulmonary Artery (1 cm distal of the Pulmonary Artery Valve).

Flow occurs in the diastole phase and is directed away from the transducer and below the Baseline. The flow, in contrast to the aortic, has a small amplitude.

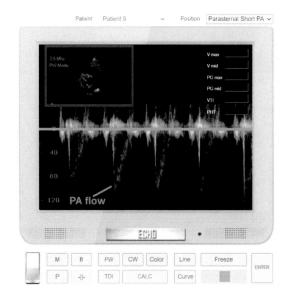

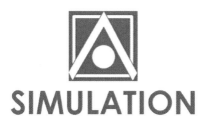

SIMULATION
PULMONARY ARTERY FLOW PW AND CW
Doppler
Echocardiography Online Simulator
MyEchocardiography.com

- Go to the link https://simulation.myechocardiography.com/

- Run Echocardiography Online Simulator using the **On/Off** Button

- Choose the patient from the list **<<Patient>>** Patient [Patient 1 ∨]

- Switch Echocardiography Simulator to **B-Mode** [B]   * *Initially Simulator is set to B-Mode.*

- Choose the position **"Parasternal Short PA"** from the list **<<Positions>>** Position [Parasternal Short PA ∨]
  or Find the position with the 3D Transducer.

- Click the button **<<PW>>** to move to Pulse Wave Spectral Doppler (PW) or **<<CW>>** to move to Continuous Wave Spectral Doppler (CW)

- Place **Sample Volume** in the Pulmonary Artery and **click.**

- To change the patient, click the **On/Off** Button

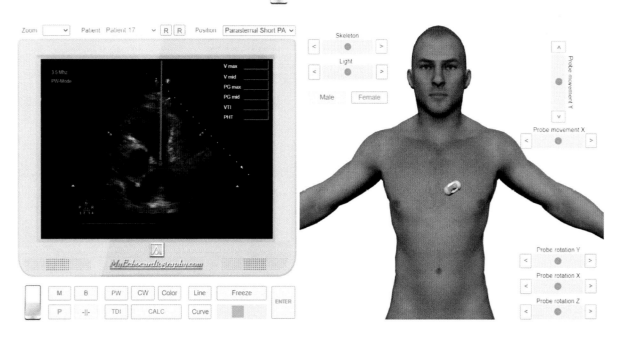

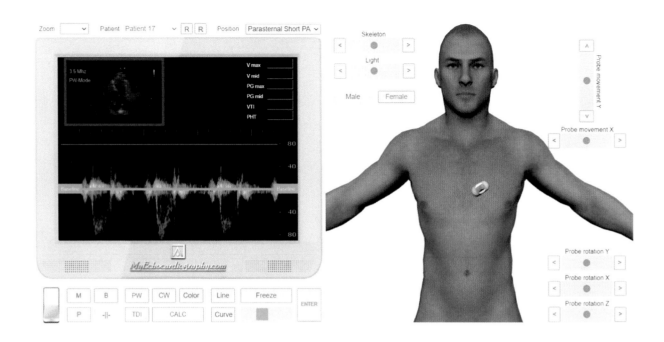

https://youtu.be/i4Fl73Yd7x4

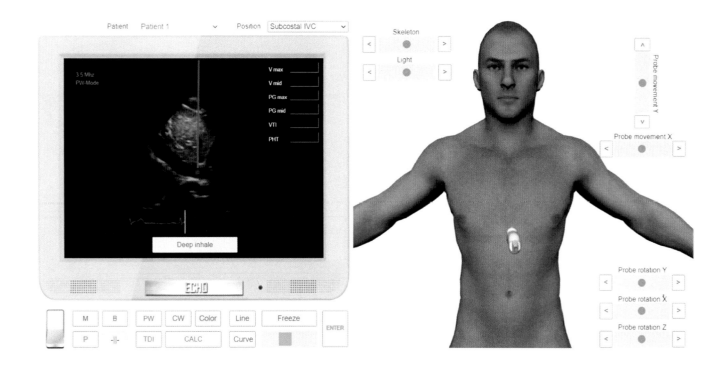

SPECTRAL DOPPLER (PW, CW)

IVC AND HEPATIC VEINS FLOW SPECTRAL

The study is carried out from a Subcostal approach, the long axis of the Inferior Vena Cava. The control volume is placed in IVC or the hepatic vein 1-2 cm proximally from its junction with the inferior vena cava.

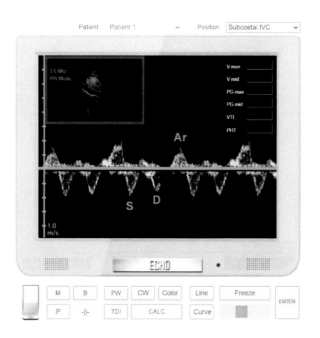

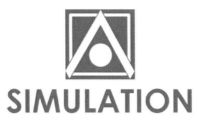

SIMULATION
IVC AND HEPATIC VEINS FLOW PW AND CW Doppler

Echocardiography Online Simulator
MyEchocardiography.com

- Go to the link https://simulation.myechocardiography.com/

- Run Echocardiography Online Simulator using the **On/Off** Button

- Choose the patient from the list **<<Patient>>** Patient [Patient 1 ⌄]

- Switch Echocardiography Simulator to **B-Mode** [B]   * Initially Simulator is set to B-Mode.

- Choose the position "**Subcostal IVC**" from the list **<<Positions>>** Position [Subcostal IVC ⌄]
  or Find the position with the 3D Transducer.

- Click the button **<<PW>>** to move to Pulse Wave Spectral Doppler (PW) or **<<CW>>** to move to Continuous Wave Spectral Doppler (CW)

- Place **Sample Volume** in the Inferior Vena Cava (IVC) and **click**.

- To change the patient, click the **On/Off** Button

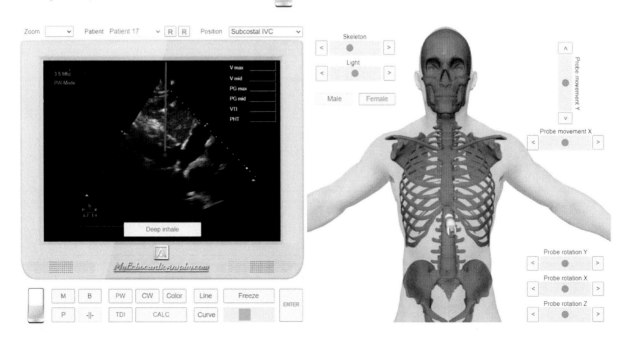

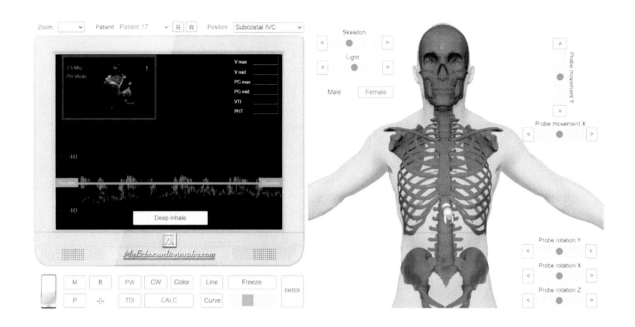

https://youtu.be/sOhzxfl5pt8

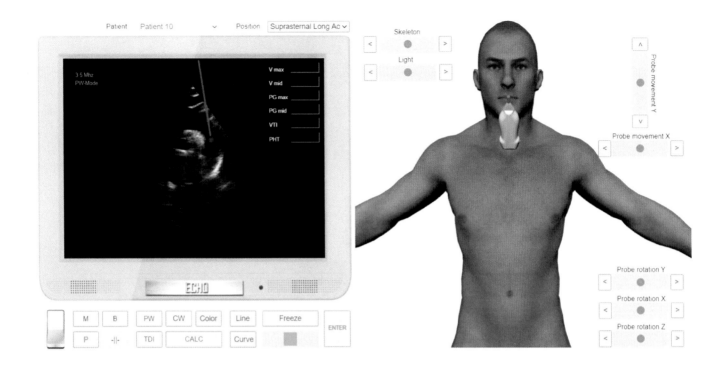

SPECTRAL DOPPLER (PW, CW)

DESCENDING AORTIC FLOW SPECTRAL DOPPLER

The study is carried out from a Suprasternal approach, the long axis of the Aorta. The control volume is placed in the Descending Aorta (1 cm distal from the left subclavian artery junction).

Typically, the flow is directed away from the transducer and located below the baseline. After the aortic arch, the velocity increases. At the end of the systole, there is a slight reversal of the flow (R).

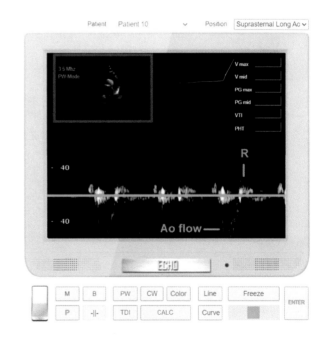

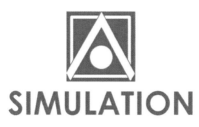

SIMULATION
DESCENDING AORTIC FLOW PW AND CW
Doppler

Echocardiography Online Simulator
MyEchocardiography.com

- Go to the link https://simulation.myechocardiography.com/

- Run Echocardiography Online Simulator using the **On/Off** Button

- Choose the patient from the list **<<Patient>>** Patient   Patient 1   ⌄

- Switch Echocardiography Simulator to **B-Mode**   B   * *Initially Simulator is set to B-Mode.*

- Choose the position "**Suprasternal Long Ao**" from the list **<<Positions>>** Position   Suprasternal Long Ao ⌄
  or Find the position with the 3D Transducer.

- Click the button **<<PW>>** to move to Pulse Wave Spectral Doppler (PW) or **<<CW>>** to move to Continuous Wave Spectral Doppler (CW)

- Place **Sample Volume** in the Descending Aorta (1 cm distal from the left subclavian artery junction) and **click.**

- To change the patient, click the **On/Off** Button

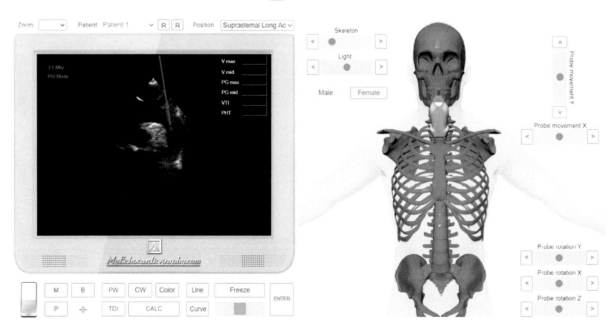

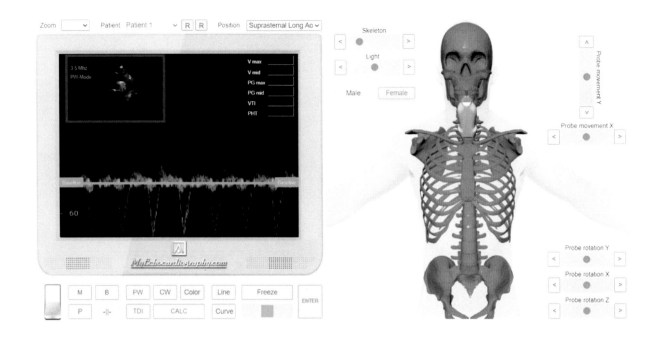

https://youtu.be/TrOP4WslYp8

COLOR DOPPLER

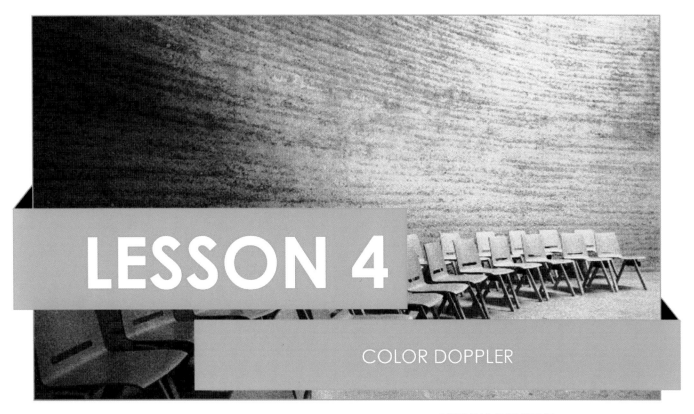

LESSON 4

COLOR DOPPLER

Color Doppler Information:

- Flow direction.
- Flow velocity.
- Flow character (laminar, turbulent)

Color Doppler:

- Trans-mitral diastolic flow Color Doppler
- Trans-tricuspid flow Color Doppler
- Left Ventricular outflow Tract (LVOT) Color Doppler
- Aortic Flow Color Doppler
- Color Doppler of the flow in the Right Ventricular Outflow Tract (RVOT) and Pulmonary Artery
- Color Doppler of the flow in Hepatic Veins and Inferior Vena Cava

Flow direction
The flow directed toward the transducer is coded in red from the transducer - in blue. Such a system is called the BART system - Blue Away, Red Toward.

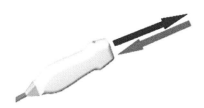

Flow velocity
Brighter blues and reds correspond to faster speeds.

Flow character (laminar, turbulent):
The laminar flow appears on the display as a homogeneous image of one color. However, the turbulent flow has a mosaic pattern and contains different colors.

COLOR DOPPLER

When examining with color Doppler, two-dimensional Echocardiography gives a two-dimensional image, and a Color Doppler superimposes the flow color-coded image on it.

Each image consists of 250 - 500 Sample Volumes oriented in a sector of the ultrasonic beam.

In the Color Doppler mode, it is essential to determine the angle between the flow and the ultrasound beam. If this angle is 90 degrees, an echo-negative space is fixed on the display - the so-called "Dead zone."

Nyquist limit = PRF/2

PRF - Pulse repetition frequency

Color Doppler Examinations

- Transmitral diastolic flow Color Doppler
- Trans-tricuspid flow Color doppler
- Left Ventricular outflow Tract (LVOT) Color Doppler
- Aortic Flow Color Doppler
- Color Doppler of the flow in the Right Ventricular Outflow Tract (RVOT) and Pulmonary Artery
- Hepatic Veins and Inferior Vena Cava flow Color Doppler

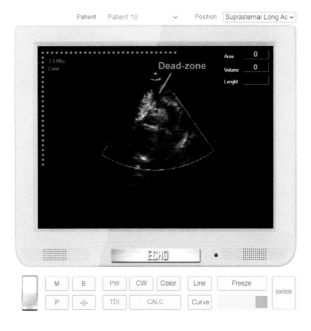

Nyquist limit

The maximum speed that can be learned in PW mode is called the Nyquist limit. If velocity is higher than this limit spectrum will be distorted. The same happens in color Doppler mode. A spectrum distortion is observed if the flow rate exceeds the Nyquist limit (colors indicate the opposite flow direction).

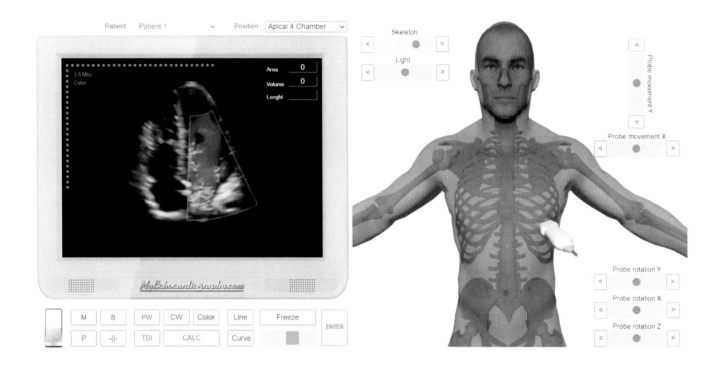

COLOR DOPPLER

TRANS-MITRAL DIASTOLIC FLOW

The best position to study trans-mitral diastolic flow by Color Doppler is the Apical 4-chamber view. In this case, the flow is more parallel to the ultrasonic beam.

Other positions from which the study can be done:

- Apical 2-chamber views.
- Left parasternal approach, the long axis of the heart.
- Subcostal 4-chamber view.

Normal trans-mitral flow occurs only in the diastole phase, is directed towards the transducer, and is encoded in red color.

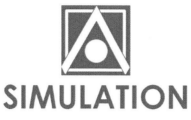

SIMULATION
TRANS-MITRAL DIASTOLIC COLOR DOPPLER

Echocardiography Online Simulator
MyEchocardiography.com

- Go to the link https://simulation.myechocardiography.com/

- Run Echocardiography Online Simulator using the **On/Off** Button

- Choose the patient from the list **<<Patient>>** Patient | Patient 1 ⌄ |

- Choose position " **Apical 4 Chamber**" from the List **<<Positions>>** Position | Apical 4 Chamber ⌄ |

or Find the position with the 3D Transducer.

- Click the Button **<<Color>>** | Color |

- To change the patient, click the **On/Off** Button

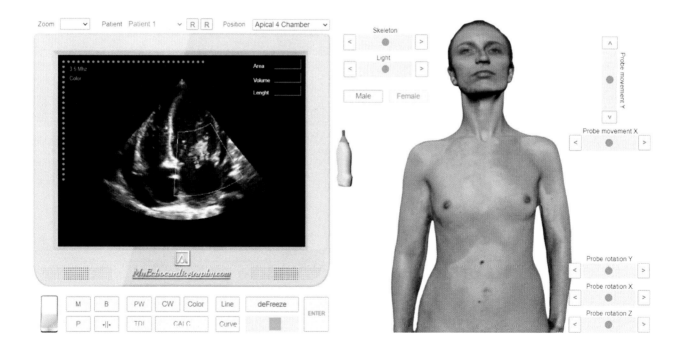

https://youtu.be/UglNlOQdANM

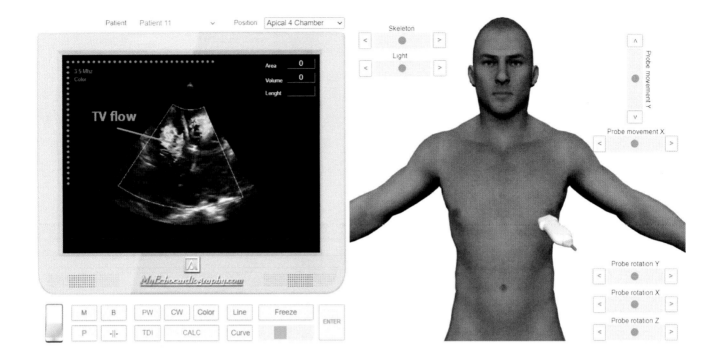

COLOR DOPPLER

TRANS-TRICUSPID DIASTOLIC FLOW

The best position to study trans-tricuspid diastolic flow by Color Doppler is the Apical 4 chamber view. In this case, the flow is more parallel to the ultrasonic beam.

The Color Doppler study can also be done from the Subcostal Four-Chamber view.

Normal trans-mitral flow occurs only in the diastole phase, is directed towards the transducer, and is encoded in red color.

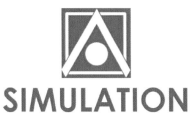

SIMULATION

TRANS-TRICUSPID DIASTOLIC FLOW COLOR DOPPLER

Echocardiography Online Simulator

MyEchocardiography.com

- Go to the link https://simulation.myechocardiography.com/

- Run Echocardiography Online Simulator using the **On/Off** Button

- Choose the patient from the list **<<Patient>>**   Patient | Patient 1   ⌄ |

- Choose position " **Apical 4 Chamber**" from the List **<<Positions>>**   Position | Apical 4 Chamber   ⌄ |

or Find the position with the 3D Transducer.

- Click the Button **<<Color>>** | Color |

- To change the patient, click the **On/Off** Button

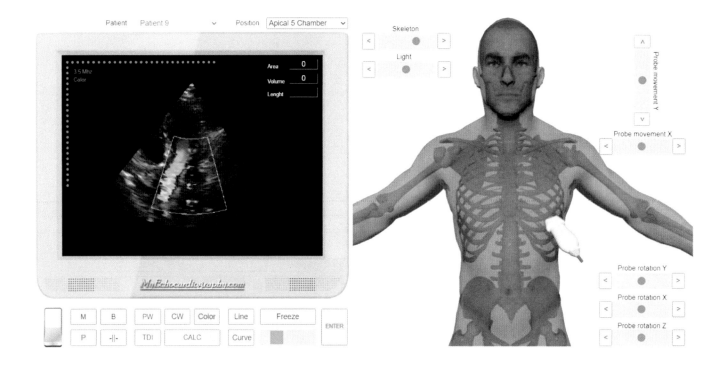

COLOR DOPPLER

LEFT VENTRICULAR OUTFLOW TRACT (LVOT) FLOW COLOR DOPPLER

The apical five-chamber position is the best choice for studying Left Ventricular Outflow Tract flow by Color Doppler. In this position, the flow is almost parallel to the ultrasonic beam. It is also possible to use the left parasternal approach, the long axis of the heart.

Normally, the flow in the outflow tract of the left ventricle occurs in the systole phase and is directed toward the aorta.

If examining from Apical 5 Chamber View, The flow is directed away from the transducer accordingly encoded in blue.

The flow will almost always exceed the Nyquist limit and is similar to the flow in the opposite direction (Spectrum Distortion).

When examining from a parasternal approach, the long axis of the heart, the flow in the left ventricular outflow tract can be directed toward the transducer or away - depending on the orientation of the outflow tract to the ultrasound beam.

If the outflow tract is in front of the transducer, then the flow is directed toward the transducer and accordingly coded in red.

When positioned at the back, the flow is directed away from the transducer and coded in blue.

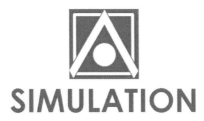

SIMULATION
LEFT VENTRICULAR OUTFLOW TRACT FLOW COLOR DOPPLER

Echocardiography Online Simulator
MyEchocardiography.com

- Go to the link https://simulation.myechocardiography.com/

- Run Echocardiography Online Simulator using the **On/Off** Button

- Choose the patient from the list **<<Patient>>** Patient | Patient 1   ∨ |

- Choose position **"Apical 5 Chamber"** or **"Parasternal Long"** from the List **<<Positions>>**
or Find the position with the 3D Transducer.

- Click the Button **<<Color>>** | Color |

- To change the patient, click the **On/Off** Button

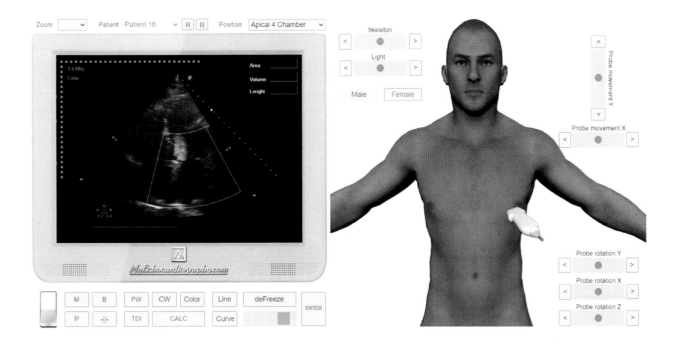

https://youtu.be/fnjeb0ZiSFU

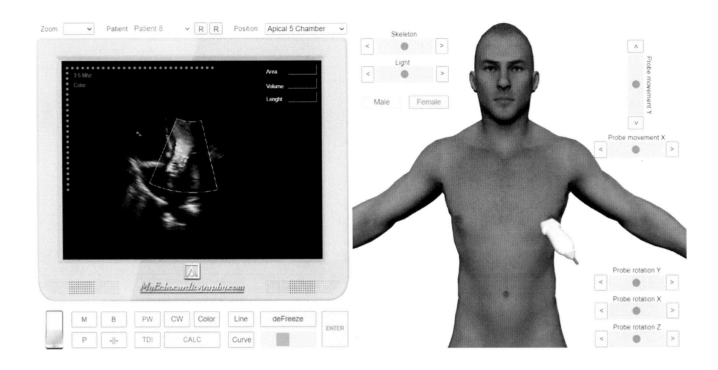

COLOR DOPPLER

AORTIC FLOW

The apical five-chamber position is the best choice for studying the flow in Ascending Aorta by Color Doppler. In this position, the flow is almost parallel to the ultrasonic beam. It is also possible to use the left parasternal approach, the long axis of the heart, And the Suprasternal View, the Long Axis of the aorta.

If examining from Apical 5 Chamber View, The flow is directed away from the transducer accordingly encoded in blue.

The flow will almost always exceed the Nyquist limit and is similar to the flow in the opposite direction (Spectrum Distortion).

When examining from a Parasternal Approach, the long axis of the heart, the flow in the Aorta can be directed towards the transducer or away from the transducer - depending on the orientation of the Aorta to the ultrasound beam.

If the Aorta is in front of the transducer, then the flow is directed toward the transducer and accordingly coded in red. When positioned at the back, the flow is directed away from the transducer and coded in blue.

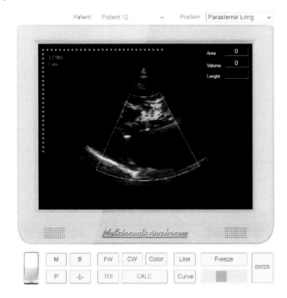

When examining Ascending aortic flow from a Suprasternal View, the flow is coded in red because it is directed toward the transducer. However, in the descending part of the aorta, it is coded in blue because it is directed away from the transducer.

In the central part, we see an echo-negative space, the so-called "dead zone." The flow in this area is perpendicular to the ultrasonic beam and cannot be investigated.

From the Subcostal View, it is possible to study flow in Abdominal Aorta. The flow is coded in red because it is directed toward the transducer.

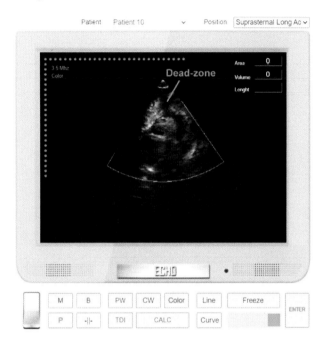

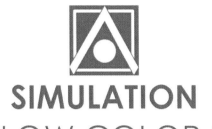

SIMULATION
AORTIC FLOW COLOR DOPPLER
Echocardiography Online Simulator
MyEchocardiography.com

- Go to the link https://simulation.myechocardiography.com/

- Run Echocardiography Online Simulator using the **On/Off** Button

- Choose the patient from the list **<<Patient>>**   Patient | Patient 1   ∨ |

- Choose **<<Apical 5 Chamber>>** or **<<Parasternal Long>>** or **<<Surpasternal Long Ao>>** or **<<Subcostal Ao>>** from the List <<Positions>> or Find the positions with the 3D Transducer.

- Click the Button **<<Color>>**   Color

- To change the patient, click the **On/Off** Button

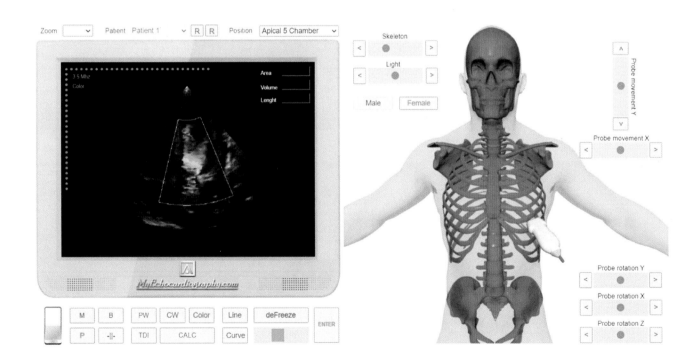

https://youtu.be/58iEUaJQSWo

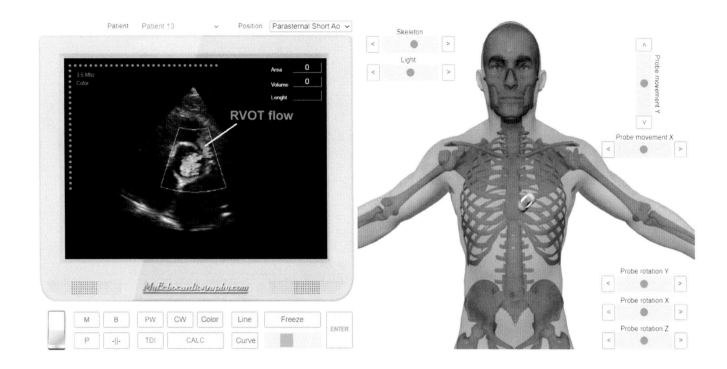

COLOR DOPPLER

RIGHT VENTRICULAR OUTFLOW TRACT (RVOT) AND PULMONARY ARTERY FLOW

Typically, the flow in the Outflow Tract of the Right Ventricle and the Pulmonary Artery is observed in the systole phase.

For studying the flow in RVOT and PA by Color Doppler, the Best positions are the Left Parasternal View, the short Axis of the heart at the level of the Aorta, and Left Parasternal View, the short Axis of the heart at the level of the pulmonary Artery.

The flow is directed away from the transducer and accordingly encoded in blue.

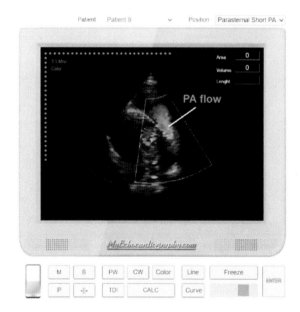

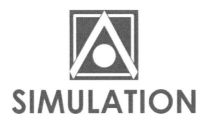

SIMULATION
RIGHT VENTRICULAR OUTFLOW TRACT (RVOT) AND PULMONARY ARTERY FLOW COLOR DOPPLER

Echocardiography Online Simulator
MyEchocardiography.com

- Go to the link https://simulation.myechocardiography.com/

- Run Echocardiography Online Simulator using the **On/Off** Button

- Choose the patient from the list **<<Patient>>** Patient Patient 1

- Choose position <<**Parasternal Short Ao>>** or **<<Parasternal Short PA>>** from the List **<<Positions>>** or Find the position with the 3D Transducer.

- Click the Button **<<Color>>** Color

- To change the patient, click the **On/Off** Button

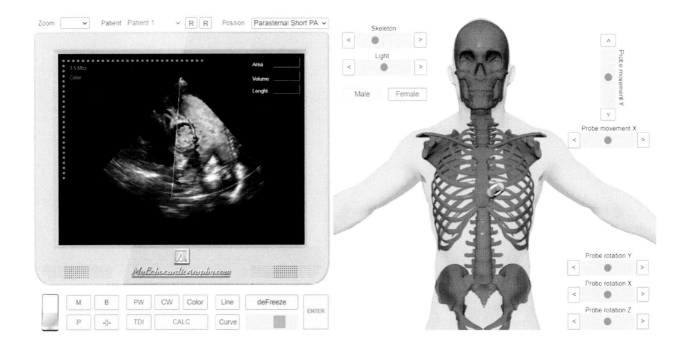

https://youtu.be/fp1u4jsUEl8

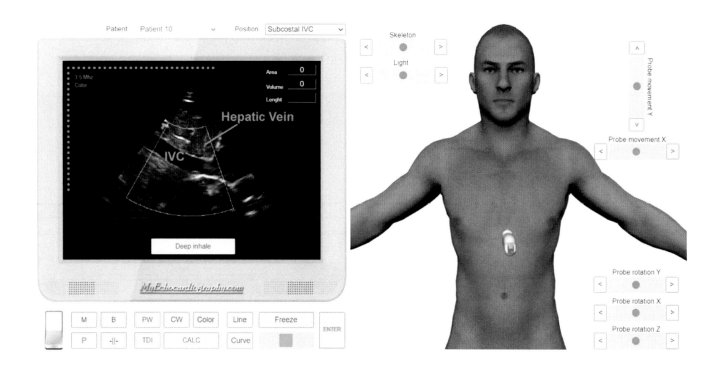

COLOR DOPPLER

INFERIOR VENA CAVA AND HEPATIC VEINS COLOR DOPPLER

The flow from the Hepatic Veins into the Inferior Vena Cava can be studied from the subcostal approach. It is directed away from the transducer and accordingly encoded in blue.

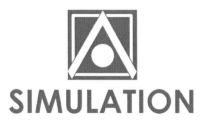

SIMULATION
INFERIOR VENA CAVA AND HEPATIC VEINS COLOR DOPPLER

Echocardiography Online Simulator
MyEchocardiography.com

- Go to the link https://simulation.myechocardiography.com/

- Run Echocardiography Online Simulator using the **On/Off** Button

- Choose the patient from the list **<<Patient>>**   Patient   Patient 1 ⌄

- Choose position <<**Subcostal IVC**>> from the List **<<Positions>>**   Position   Subcostal IVC ⌄

or Find the position with the 3D Transducer.

- Click the Button **<<Color>>**   Color

- To change the patient, click the **On/Off** Button

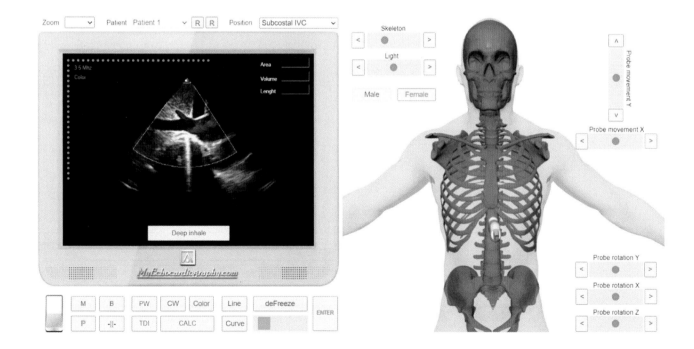

https://youtu.be/7INEE0Gem60

TISSUE DOPPLER

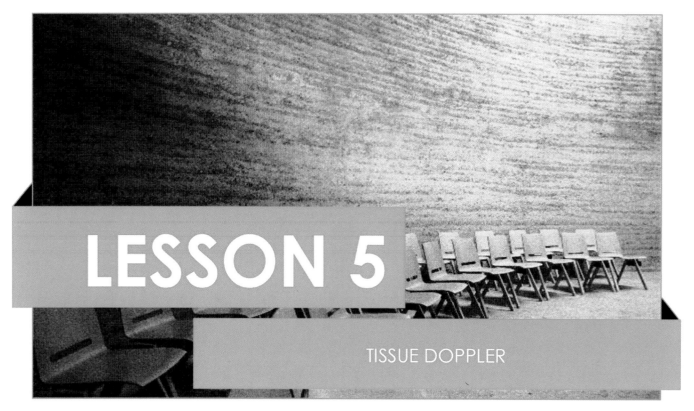

LESSON 5

TISSUE DOPPLER

The myocardium has subendocardial and epicardial layers, with the former having longitudinally arranged myofibres. During ventricular contraction, various layers exert varying tension with the endocardium moving greater distances. Tissue Doppler imaging examines the longitudinal component of myocardial contraction throughout the cardiac cycle.

Tissue Doppler imaging is obtained using pulsed wave tissue Doppler or colour tissue Doppler imaging (CTDI).

Pulsed wave TDI measures peak longitudinal myocardial velocity from a single segment, but has to be performed 'on line'.

Colour tissue Doppler imaging is performed 'off line', and can interrogate velocities from multiple sites simultaneously.

The major disadvantage of TDI is its angle dependence i.e. if the angle of incidence exceeds 15 degrees, there is 4% underestimation of velocity. Accurate TDI imaging additionally requires high frame rates (>100fps) for image acquisition with excellent temporal resolution.

The TDI signal over a cardiac cycle has three peaks, a positive systolic peak and two negative diastolic peaks. The positive systolic wave (s' velocity, Sa or Sm) represents myocardial contraction.

The negative waves represent the early diastolic myocardial relaxation (e' velocity, Ea or Em) and active atrial contraction in late diastole (a' velocity, Aa or Am).

LESSON CONTENT

Tissue Doppler:

- Septal and Lateral Tissue Doppler
- Simulation of the Septal and Lateral Tissue Doppler

TISSUE DOPPLER

Septal and Lateral Tissue Doppler

Pulsed wave TDI velocity measurements are obtained by placing the sample volume at the mitral annular level (denoted Sa/s' or Ea/e' or Aa/a') or within the basal LV myocardial segment (denoted Sm or Em or Am).

Tissue Doppler imaging velocities can be measured either from the septal or lateral annulus, but the current recommendation is that e' velocity is expressed as the average of septal and lateral measurements.

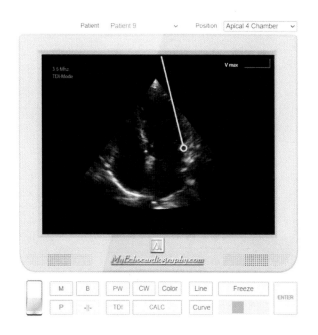

Apical 4 chamber view. Sample Volume position for the Lateral TDI. Simulation by Echocardiography Online Simulator MyEchocardiography.com

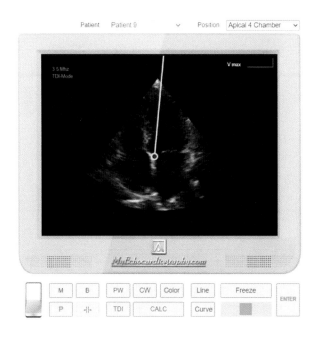

Apical 4 chamber view. Sample Volume position for the Septal TDI. Simulation by Echocardiography Online Simulator MyEchocardiography.com

Echocardiography Online Simulator MyEchocardiography.com allows simulation of Pulsed wave TDI in Apical 4 Chamber View at the mitral annular level (Septal and Lateral).

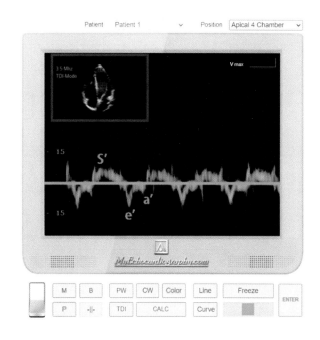

Tissue Doppler (TDI). S' - The positive systolic wave represents myocardial contraction. e' - early diastolic myocardial relaxation. a' - active atrial contraction in late diastole. Simulation by Echocardiography Online Simulator MyEchocardiography.com

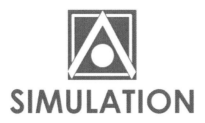

SIMULATION
SEPTAL AND LATERAL TISSUE DOPPLER
Echocardiography Online Simulator
MyEchocardiography.com

- Go to the link https://simulation.myechocardiography.com/

- Run Echocardiography Online Simulator using the **On/Off** Button

- Choose the patient from the list **<<Patient>>** Patient Patient 1 ⌄

- Choose position " **Apical 4 Chamber**" from the List **<<Positions>>** Position Apical 4 Chamber ⌄

or Find the position with the 3D Transducer.

- Click the Button **<<TDI>>** TDI

- Plase the Sample Volume at the Motral Annular level (Septal or Lateral) and Click.

- To change the patient, click the **On/Off** Button

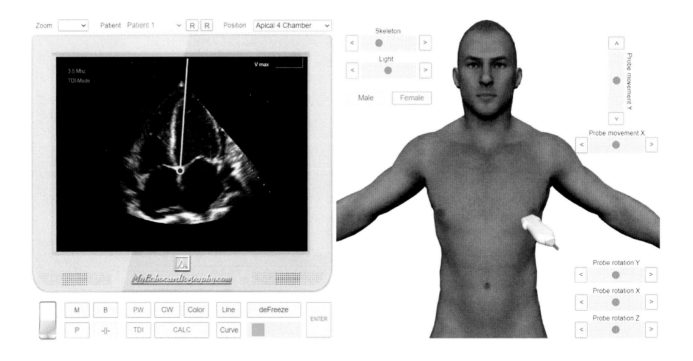

https://youtu.be/qe0r5B1t6ks

ECHOCARDIOGRAPHY

MEASUREMENTS

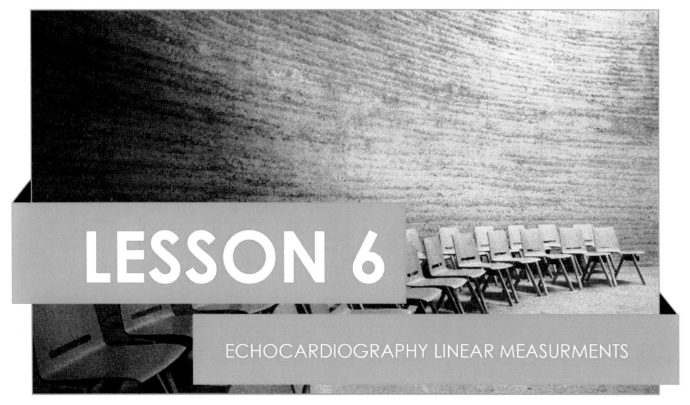

LESSON 6

ECHOCARDIOGRAPHY LINEAR MEASURMENTS

2D echocardiography enables real-time visualization of heart structures, performing different measurements and calculations.

The American Society of Echocardiography recommends measurement standards.

Various factors can distort the accuracy of measurements and calculations.

Image Quality depends on the ultrasonic instrument and transducer frequency. Therefore, the optimal image is obtained using the highest frequency that provides the desired penetration.

For accurate measurements, obtaining a clear image of the endocardium is important.

Linear measurements of the heart chambers and big vessels:

- Linear measurements of the left ventricle
- Linear measurements of the right ventricle
- Linear measurements of the Mitral and Tricuspid Annulus
- Linear measurements of the Left and Right Ventricle Outflow Tract
- Linear measurements of the left and right atrium
- Linear measurements of the Aorta
- Linear measurements of the Pulmonary Artery
- Linear Measurement of the Inferior Vena Cava and Hepatic Veins

LESSON CONTENT

Linear Measurements:

- Linear measurements of the left ventricle
- Linear measurements of the right ventricle
- Linear measurements of the Mitral and Tricuspid Annulus
- Linear measurements of the Left and Right Ventricle Outflow Tract
- Linear measurements of the left and right atrium
- Linear measurements of the Aorta
- Linear measurements of the Pulmonary Artery
- Linear Measurement of the Inferior Vena Cava and Hepatic Veins

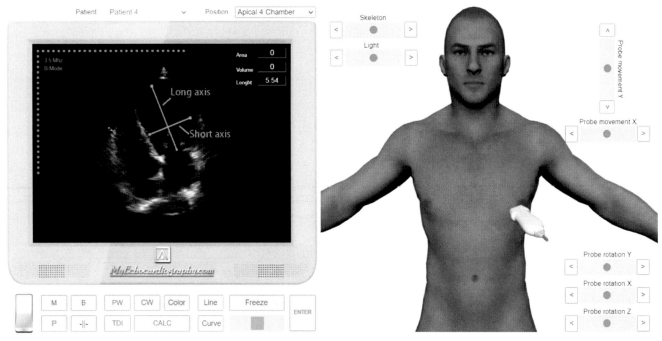

Apical 4 Chamber view. Linear measurements of the Left Ventricle. Simulation By Echocardiography Online Simulator MyEchocardiography.com

LINEAR MEASURMENTS

LINEAR MEASURMENTS OF THE LEFT VENTRICLE

The long axis of the left ventricle can be measured from the Apical Four-chamber and Two-chamber positions. Measurements are taken from the endocardium of the Apex to the center of the mitral annulus. In the Left Parasternal position, the Apex of the heart is not visualized, so it is impossible to use this position to measure the long axis.

The short axis of the left ventricle can be measured in the Apical Four-chamber position and various positions from the parasternal approach. In the Apical Four-chamber view, measurements are taken perpendicular to the long axis of the left ventricle. The hypothetical long axis is divided into three equal parts, and measurements are taken along the line that passes at the closest point from the mitral annulus.

The short axis of the left ventricle can also be measured from the Left Parasternal Approach, the Long and Short axis of the heart. In this case, the short axis is measured perpendicular to the long axis at the level of the ends of the mitral valve leaflets.

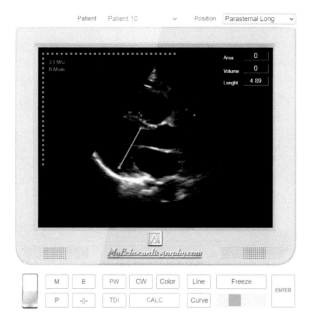

Apical 4 Chamber view. Linear measurements of the Left Ventricle. Simulation By Echocardiography Online Simulator MyEchocardiography.com

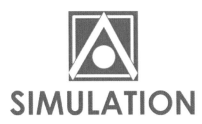

SIMULATION
LINEAR MEASURMENTS OF THE LEFT VENTRICLE

Echocardiography Online Simulator
MyEchocardiography.com

- Go to the link https://simulation.myechocardiography.com/

- Run Echocardiography Online Simulator using the **On/Off** Button

- Choose the patient from the list **<<Patient>>** Patient   Patient 1   ⌄

- Choose position <<**Apical 4 Chamber**>> or <<**Apical 2 Chamber**>> or <<**Parasternal Long**>> from the List

  <<Positions>> or find the position with the 3D Transducer.

- Click the Button **<<Line>>** Line and perform the linear measurements.

- To change the patient, click the **On/Off** Button

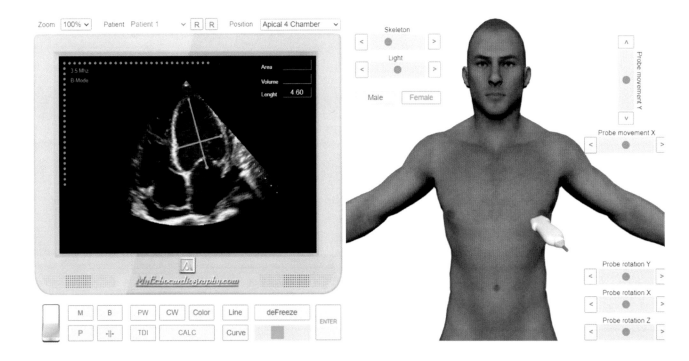

https://youtu.be/2Ht5_nefk9k

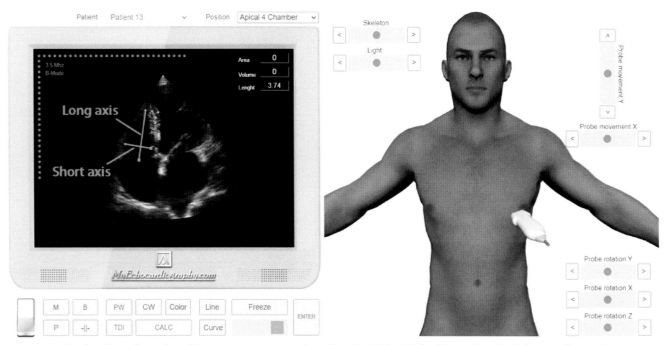

Apical 4 Chamber view. Linear measurements of the Right Ventricle. Simulation By Echocardiography Online Simulator MyEchocardiography.com

LINEAR MEASURMENTS

LINEAR MEASURMENTS OF THE RIGHT VENTRICLE

The long and short axis of the Right Ventricle can be measured from the Apical four-chamber view. The long axis is measured from the endocardium of the apex to the center of the mitral annulus.

For the measurement of the short axis, the hypothetical long axis is divided into three equal parts, and measurements are taken along the line that passes at the closest point from the mitral annulus.

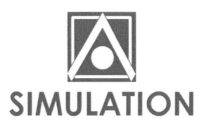

SIMULATION
LINEAR MEASURMENTS OF THE RIGHT VENTRICLE

Echocardiography Online Simulator
MyEchocardiography.com

- Go to the link https://simulation.myechocardiography.com/

- Run Echocardiography Online Simulator using the **On/Off** Button

- Choose the patient from the list **<<Patient>>**   Patient | Patient 1 ∨ |

- Choose position <<**Apical 4 Chamber**>> from the List **<<Positions>>** or find the position with the 3D

  Transducer.

- Click the Button **<<Line>>** | Line | and perform the linear measurements.

- To change the patient, click the **On/Off** Button

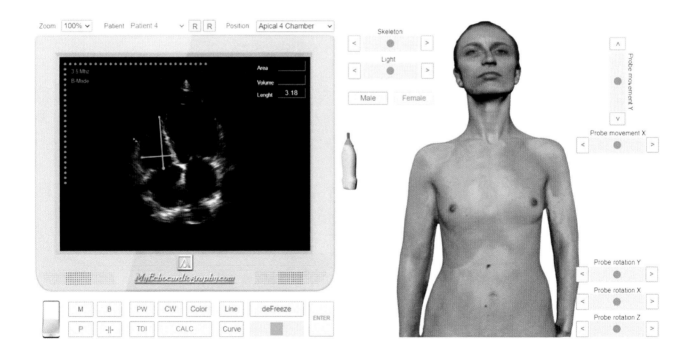

https://youtu.be/5LkVSQajYxg

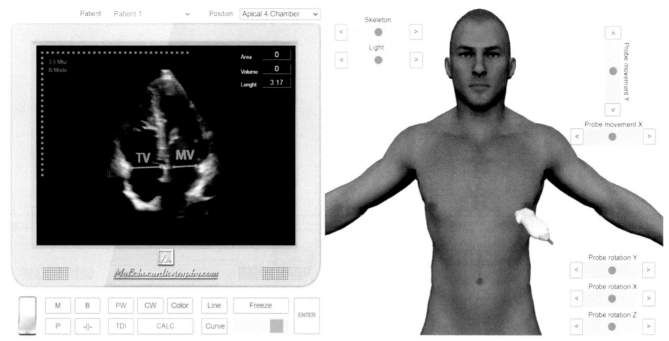

Apical 4 Chamber view. Linear measurements of the Mitral and Tricuspid Annulus. Simulation By Echocardiography Online Simulator MyEchocardiography.com

LINEAR MEASURMENTS

MITRAL AND TRICUSPID ANNULUS LINEAR MEASUREMENTS

Linear measurements of the Mitral Annulus can be performed from the Apical 4 Chamber View and Apical 2 chamber view in the middle phase of diastole.

Linear measurements of the Tricuspid Annulus can be performed from the Apical 4 Chamber View in the middle phase of the diastole.

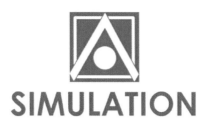

SIMULATION
MITRAL AND TRICUSPID ANNULUS LINEAR MEASUREMENTS

Echocardiography Online Simulator
MyEchocardiography.com

- Go to the link https://simulation.myechocardiography.com/

- Run Echocardiography Online Simulator using the **On/Off** Button

- Choose the patient from the list **<<Patient>>**   Patient   Patient 1   ⌄

- Choose position <<**Apical 4 Chamber**>> from the List **<<Positions>>** or find the position with the 3D

  Transducer.

- Click the Button **<<Line>>** Line and perform the linear measurements.

- To change the patient, click the **On/Off** Button

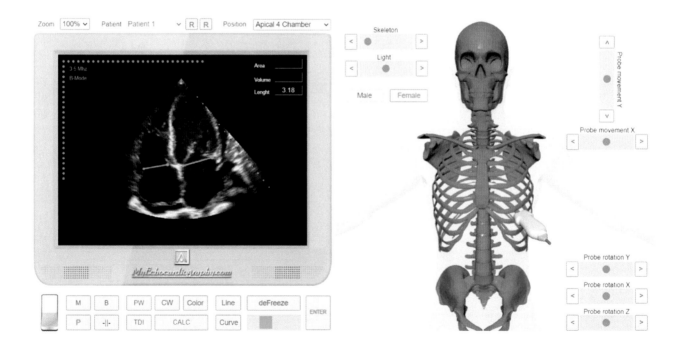

https://youtu.be/G5hHLtLyQtE

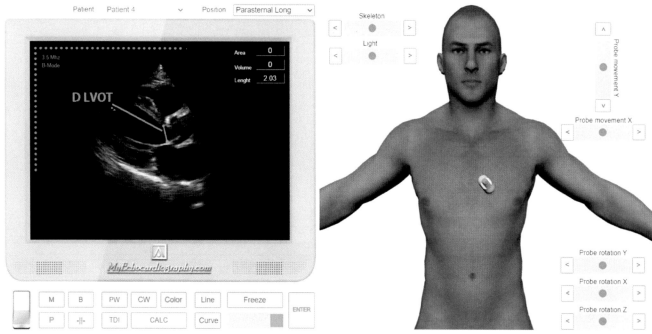

Left Parasternal View, the Long axis. Linear measurements of the Left Ventricle Outflow Tract. Simulation By Echocardiography Online Simulator MyEchocardiography.com

LINEAR MEASURMENTS

LVOT AND RVOT LINEAR MEASUREMENTS

In the systole phase, the outflow tract of the left ventricle (LVOT) is measured from the Parasternal View, the Long Axis of the heart. Measurement has to be done from the inner edge of the junction of the anterior wall of the aorta with the interventricular septum to the inner edge of the junction of the posterior wall of the aorta with the anterior leaflet of the mitral valve (0.5 -1 cm from the Ao valve in the left ventricle).

Measurement of the right ventricular outflow tract (RVOT) is performed from the Left parasternal View, the short axis, at the level of the Aortic Valve in the systole phase, proximal of the Pulmonary Valve (0.5 -1 cm from the PA valve in the right ventricle).

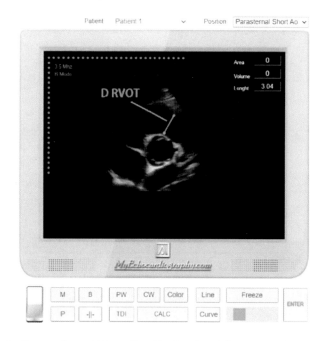

Left parasternal View, the Short axis, at the level of the Aortic Valve. Linear measurements of the Right Ventricle Outflow Tract. Simulation By Echocardiography Online Simulator MyEchocardiography.com

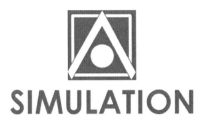

SIMULATION
LVOT AND RVOT LINEAR MEASUREMENTS
Echocardiography Online Simulator
MyEchocardiography.com

- Go to the link https://simulation.myechocardiography.com/

- Run Echocardiography Online Simulator using the **On/Off** Button

- Choose the patient from the list **<<Patient>>**   Patient   Patient 1   ⌄

- Choose position <<**Parasternal Long**>> or <<**Parasternal Short Ao>>** or <<**Parasternal Short PA>>** from the List <<**Positions>>** or find the position with the 3D Transducer.

- Click the Button <<**Line>>**   Line   and perform the linear measurements.

- To change the patient, click the **On/Off** Button .

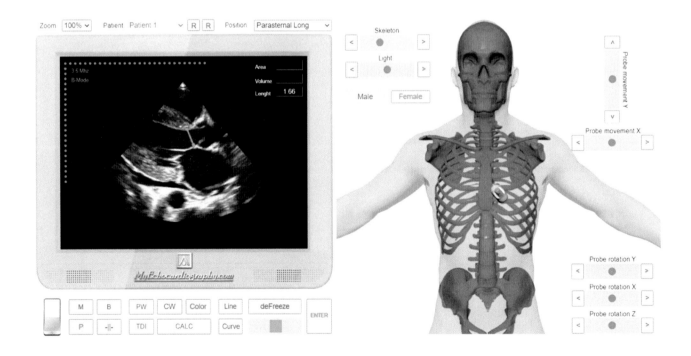

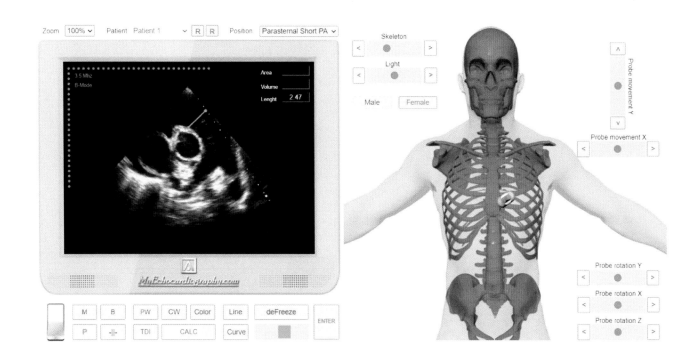

https://youtu.be/mj8VoBhNzGs

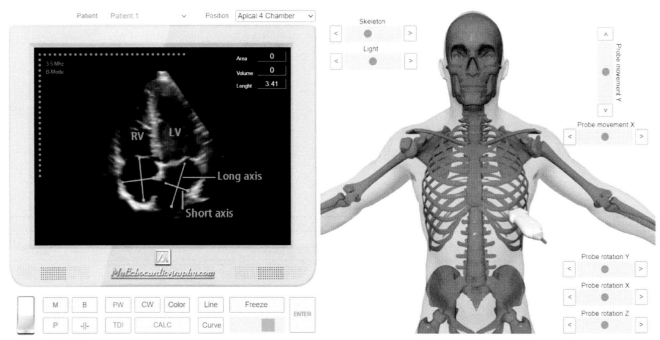

Left Parasternal View, the Long axis. Linear measurements of Left and Right Atriums. Simulation By Echocardiography Online Simulator MyEchocardiography.com

LINEAR MEASURMENTS

LEFT AND RIGHT ATRIUM LINEAR MEASUREMENTS

The long and short axis of the Left Atrium can be measured from the Apical four-chamber view, Apical two-chamber view, Left Parasternal view, Long axis, and Short axis at the level of the Aorta.
The long and short axis of the Right Atrium can be measured from the Apical four-chamber view.

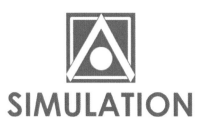

SIMULATION
LEFT AND RIGHT ATRIUM LINEAR MEASUREMENTS

Echocardiography Online Simulator
MyEchocardiography.com

- Go to the link https://simulation.myechocardiography.com/

- Run Echocardiography Online Simulator using the **On/Off** Button

- Choose the patient from the list **<<Patient>>** Patient Patient 1 ⌄

- Choose position **<<Apical 4 Chamber>>** or find the position with the 3D Transducer.

- Click the Button **<<Line>>** Line and perform the linear measurements.

- To change the patient, click the **On/Off** Button .

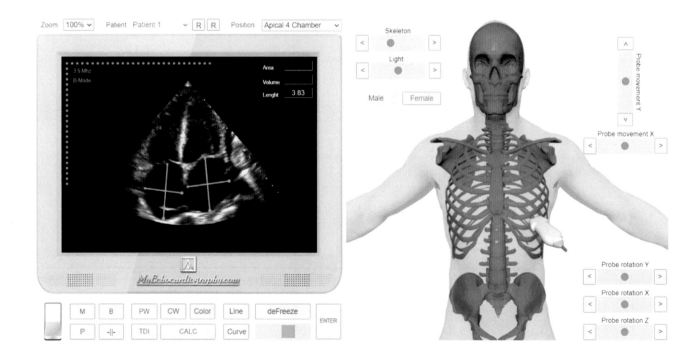

https://youtu.be/Ddmde_dNUO8

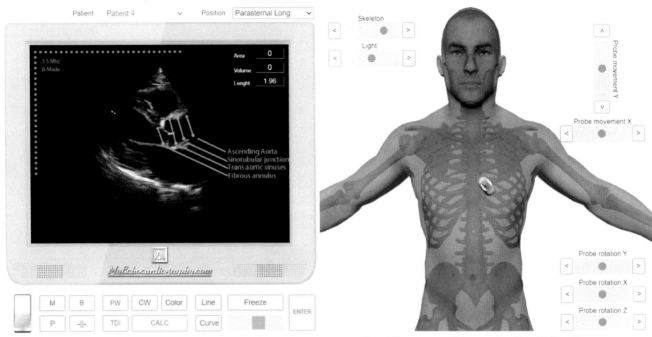

Left Parasternal view. Long axis. Linear measurements of the Ascending Aorta. Simulation By Echocardiography Online Simulator MyEchocardiography.com

LINEAR MEASURMENTS

LINEAR MEASUREMENTS OF THE AORTA

Aorta can be measured at different levels:

- The fibrous annulus of the aorta **(AoA)**
- Transaortic sinuses **(AoSV)**
- Sinotubular junction **(AoSTJ)**
- Proximal ascending aorta diameter **(AoPxA)**
- Aortic arch **(AoArch)**
- Descending aorta **(AoDesc)**
- Abdominal aorta **(AoAbd)**

Determining the linear sizes of the Aorta at the level of the Annulus, Transaortic Sinuses, Ascending Aorta, and Sinotubular junction is possible from the Left Parasternal view, Long axis.

The Transaortic Sinuses can also be measured from the Left Parasternal view, the Short axis at the Aortic Valve level.

The Aortic arch and Descending Aorta are measured from the Suprasternal Approach.

From the Subcostal Approach, it is possible to measure the Linear Size of the Abdominal Aorta.

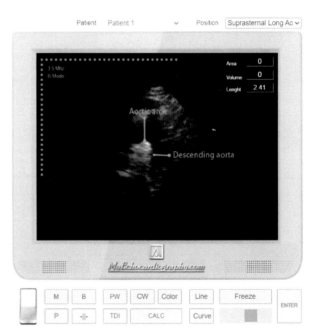

Suprasternal view. The long axis of the Aorta. Linear measurements of the Aortic arch and descending Aorta. Simulation By Echocardiography Online Simulator MyEchocardiography.com

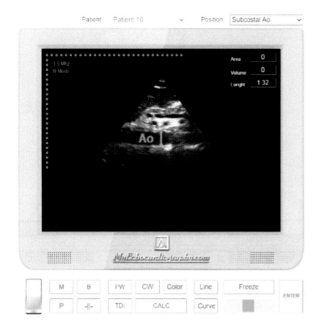

Subcostal view of the Abdominal Aorta. Linear measurements of the Abdominal Aorta. Simulation By Echocardiography Online Simulator MyEchocardiography.com

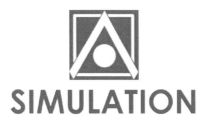

SIMULATION
LINEAR MEASUREMENTS OF THE AORTA

Echocardiography Online Simulator
MyEchocardiography.com

- Go to the link https://simulation.myechocardiography.com/

- Run Echocardiography Online Simulator using the **On/Off** Button

- Choose the patient from the list **<<Patient>>** Patient   Patient 1   ∨

- Choose position **<<Parasternal Long>>** or **<<Parasternal Short Ao>>** or **<<Parasternal Short PA>>** from

  the List **<<Positions>>** or find the position with the 3D Transducer.

- Click the Button **<<Line>>** Line and perform the linear measurements.

- To change the patient, click the **On/Off** Button .

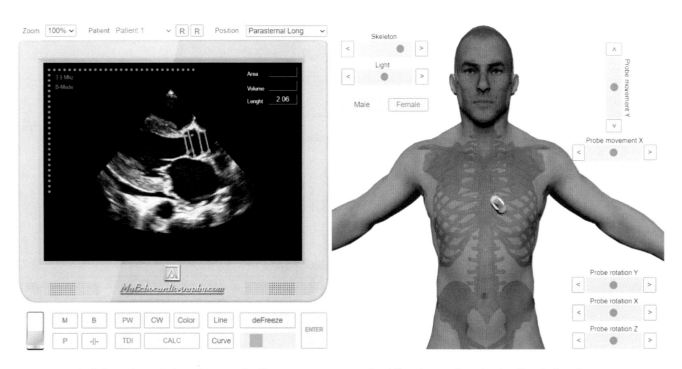

Left Parasternal view. Long axis. Linear measurements of the Ascending Aorta. Simulation By
Echocardiography Online Simulator MyEchocardiography.com

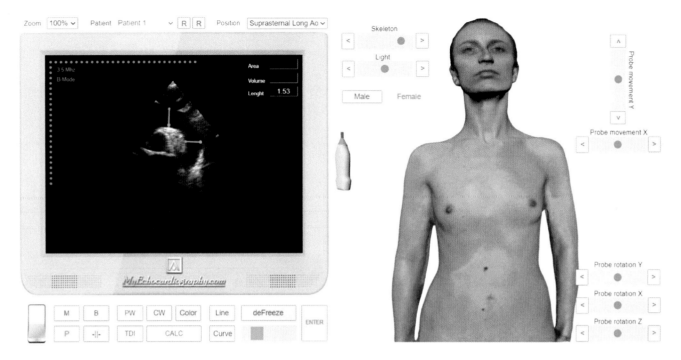

Suprasternal view. The long axis of the Aorta. Linear measurements of the Aortic arch and descending Aorta. Simulation By Echocardiography Online Simulator MyEchocardiography.com

https://youtu.be/HlAbGVnIfFE

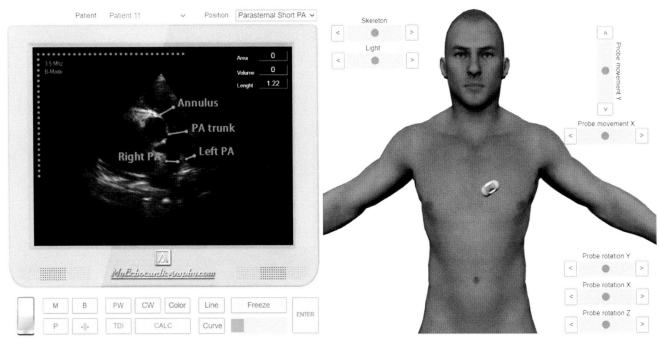

*Left Parasternal View, the long axis of Pulmonary Artery. Linear measurements of Pulmonary Artery.
Simulation By Echocardiography Online Simulator MyEchocardiography.com*

LINEAR MEASURMENTS

PULMONARY ARTERY LINEAR MEASUREMENTS

Pulmonary Valve Annulus, Pulmonary Artery trunk, and Left and Right Pulmonary Arteries can be measured from the Left Parasternal View, the long axis of the Pulmonary Artery.

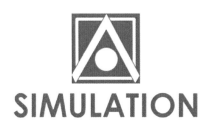

SIMULATION
PULMONARY ARTERY LINEAR MEASUREMENTS

Echocardiography Online Simulator
MyEchocardiography.com

- Go to the link https://simulation.myechocardiography.com/

- Run Echocardiography Online Simulator using the **On/Off** Button

- Choose the patient from the list **<<Patient>>** Patient Patient 1

- Choose position <<**Parasternal Short PA**>> from the List **<<Positions>>** or find the position with the 3D

  Transducer.

- Click the Button **<<Line>>** Line and perform the linear measurements.

- To change the patient, click the **On/Off** Button

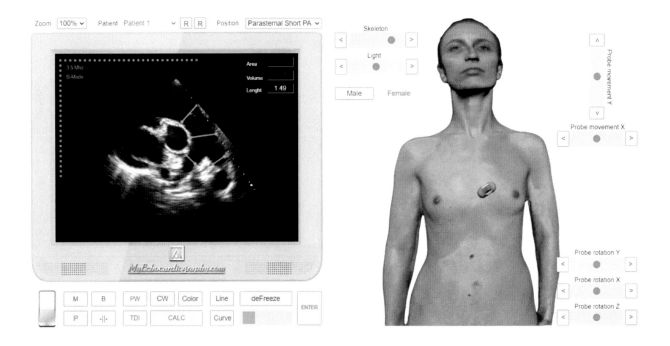

https://youtu.be/Owv8JMeBScs

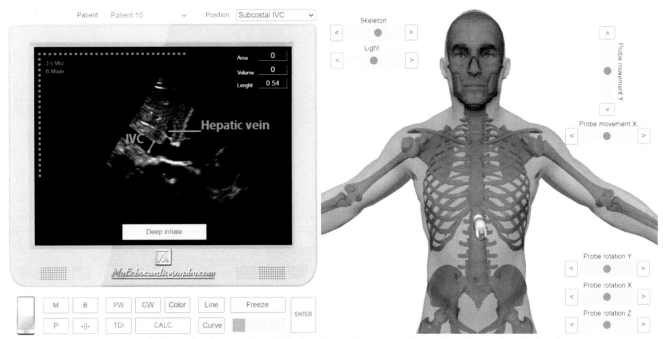

Patient Patient 10 ⌄ Position Subcostal IVC ⌄

Area 0
Volume 0
Lenght 0.54

3.5 Mhz
B-Mode

Hepatic vein

IVC

Deep inhale

MyEchocardiography.com

M B PW CW Color Line Freeze
P -||- TDI CALC Curve ENTER

Skeleton < ● >
Light < ● >

Probe movement Y ∧ ● ∨
Probe movement X < ● >

Probe rotation Y < ● >
Probe rotation X < ● >
Probe rotation Z < ● >

Subcostal View, the long axis of Inferior Vena Cava and Hepatic Veins. Simulation By Echocardiography Online Simulator MyEchocardiography.com

LINEAR MEASURMENTS

INFERIOR VENA CAVA AND HEPATIC VEINS LINEAR MEASUREMENTS

Linear measurements of the Inferior Vena Cava and Hepatic Veins can be performed from the Subcostal View, the long axis of the Inferior Vena Cava and Hepatic Veins.

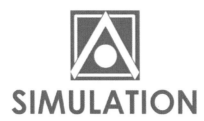

SIMULATION
INFERIOR VENA CAVA AND HEPATIC VEINS
LINEAR MEASUREMENTS
Echocardiography Online Simulator
MyEchocardiography.com

- Go to the link https://simulation.myechocardiography.com/

- Run Echocardiography Online Simulator using the **On/Off** Button

- Choose the patient from the list **<<Patient>>**   Patient   Patient 1   ⌄

- Choose position <<**Subcostal IVC**>> from the List **<<Positions>>** or find the position with the 3D

  Transducer.

- Click the Button **<<Line>>**   Line   and perform the linear measurements.

- To change the patient, click the **On/Off** Button

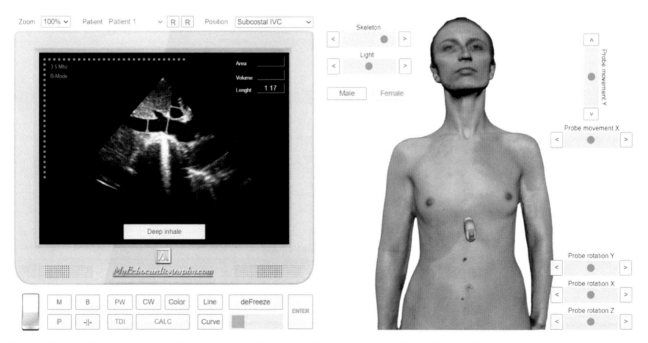

Subcostal View, the long axis of Inferior Vena Cava and Hepatic Veins. Simulation By Echocardiography Online Simulator MyEchocardiography.com

https://youtu.be/-7hNTdwCFo4

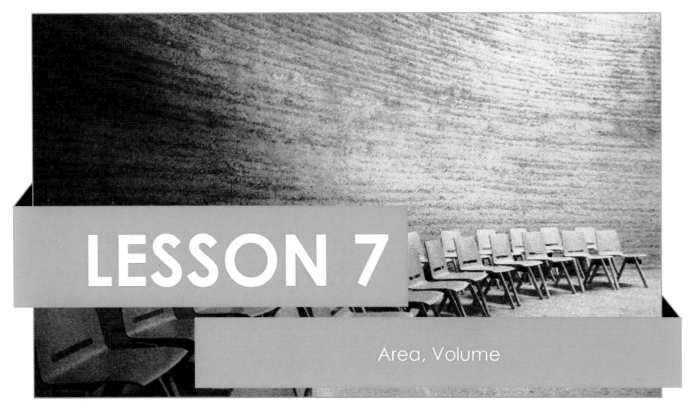

LESSON 7

Area, Volume

Calculating the area of heart structures

With two-dimensional echocardiography, it is possible to calculate the area of the following structures of the heart:

- Fibrous ring.
- Cardiac chamber.
- Valve hole.

The area is calculated using mathematical formulas embedded in the ultrasound devices, with a:

- Radius.
- Diameter.
- Circumference.

Calculating the area using the radius:

$$S = \pi r^2$$

Calculating the area using the diameter:

$$S = 0,785 \times D^2$$

Area, Volume:

- Calculating the area of heart structures.
- Calculating the volume of the heart chambers.
- Left ventricular volume.
- Right ventricular volume.
- Left and right atrial volumes.

Calculating the area using the circumference:

$$S = \left(\frac{1}{2}\right) \sum_{i-1}^{n-1} x_i(y_i - y_{i-1}) - y_i(x_i - x_{i-1})$$

Modern echocardiographs have built-in formulas for calculating the area, which allows us to automatically obtain a specific value of the desired area when we fix the radius, diameter, or circumference on the screen.

The volume of the heart chambers

With two-dimensional echocardiography, it is possible to determine the volume of the heart chambers. It is possible to calculate the systolic and diastolic volumes of the ventricles and atria.

With two-dimensional echocardiography, it is possible to determine the volume of the heart chambers. It is possible to calculate the systolic and diastolic volumes of the ventricles and atria.

Left ventricular volume

To calculate the volume of the left ventricle, its area, and linear size are used. The volume is measured in the apical four-chamber and two-chamber positions. These two positions are orthogonal to each other (60 to 90 degrees).

Two methods are recommended for calculating the volume of the left ventricle:

- Simpson's modified method (method of the discs).
- "Area-Length" method.

The volume calculation is provided by the computer program installed in the echocardiographs. The researcher traces the inner surface of the endocardium of the single ventricle.

Below is the formula used to make such calculations:

$$V = 0{,}85 \times \frac{A^2}{L}$$

The calculation of the ventricle volume by Simpson's method is based on the principle of summing up the discs. With this method, the ventricle is divided into a series of disks, and the volume of the ventricle calculated by the corresponding algorithm is close to the results obtained by angiography. The calculation of the volume with the mentioned method is provided by the computer program installed in the echocardiographs. The operator traces the inner surface of the endocardium of the single ventricle.

The length of the discs is obtained by dividing the length of the long axis of the ventricle into 20 equal segments. Disc diameters are measured in 2 orthogonal positions – Simpson's bi-plane method (apical four-chamber and two-chamber positions).

The length of the long axis should be approximately equal in both positions. While the difference between their lengths is more than 20%, the volume measurement result should not be accepted.

$$V = \frac{\pi}{4} \sum_{i=1}^{20} a_i b_i \frac{L}{20}$$

a - Disc diameter in one position

b - Diameter of the disk in the second position

L - The length of the long axis of the ventricle

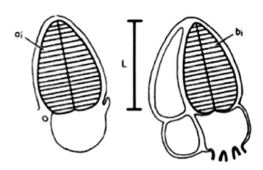

Calculation of the left ventricular volume by Simpson's bi-plane method. Left-apical two-chamber view. Right-apical four-chamber view.

Calculating the volume of the left ventricle using the "area-length" method:

This method is used when only one apical position can be obtained.

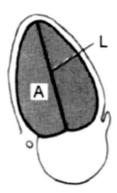

Calculation of the left ventricular volume using the Area-length method.

Right ventricular volume

Despite numerous attempts, no method has been developed to correctly calculate the right ventricular volume because of its irregular geometry and the impossibility of perfect visualization.

Therefore, right ventricular volume measurement is not performed during routine echocardiographic examination.

Atrial volume

Left and right atrial volumes are calculated when atrial volumes are maximal during ventricular systole.

The volume of the left ventricle can be calculated in the following positions:

- Apical four-chamber position.

- Apical bicameral position.

- Left parasternal position, the long axis of the heart.

- Left parasternal position, the short axis of the heart, at the level of the aortic valve.

Right atrial volume can only be calculated from the apical four-chamber position.

The volume of the atria can be calculated by the following methods:

- "Area-Length" method.
- "Discs" method.

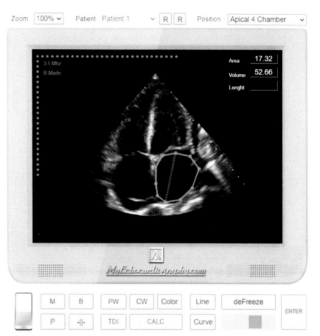

Apical 4-chamber view. Measurement of the left atrium volume. Simulation By Echocardiography Online Simulator MyEchocardiography.com

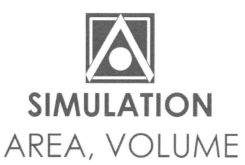

SIMULATION
AREA, VOLUME
Echocardiography Online Simulator
MyEchocardiography.com

- Go to the link https://simulation.myechocardiography.com/

- Run Echocardiography Online Simulator using the **On/Off** Button

- Choose the patient from the list **<<Patient>>**   Patient   Patient 1

- Choose a position from the List **<<Positions>>** or Find a position with the 3D Transducer.

- Click the button **<<Curve>>** place points around area of interest and Click the button **<<Enter>>**

- To change the patient, click the **On/Off** Button

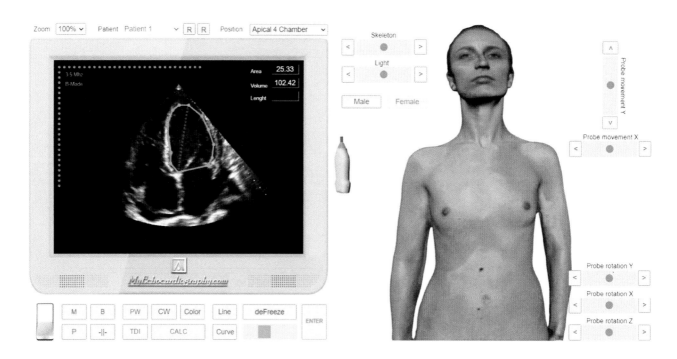

Apical 4-chamber view. Measurement of the Left Ventricular Volume. Simulation By Echocardiography Online Simulator MyEchocardiography.com

https://youtu.be/Dt9mI59ldTI

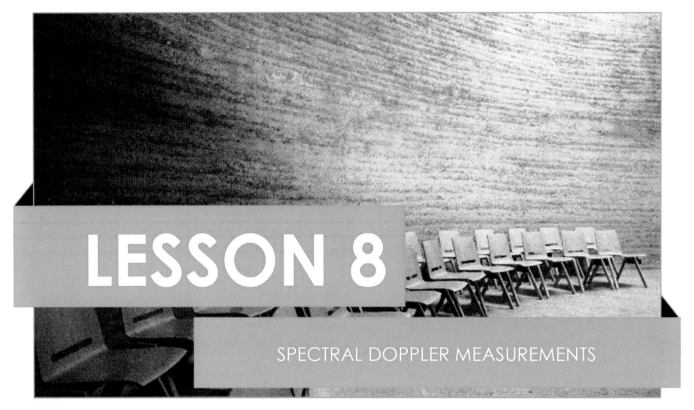

LESSON 8

SPECTRAL DOPPLER MEASUREMENTS

Vmax and Vmid

Vmax - Maximum flow velocity.
Vmid (Average Flow Velocity) - The sum of the flow velocities measured every 2 seconds, divided by the number of measurements.

PGmax and PGmid

The blood movement between the heart chambers depends on the pressure difference between the chambers. The pressure gradient can be determined using the simplified Bernoulli formula:

$$\triangle p = 4V^2$$

V - flow velosity.

PGmax - Maximum flow gradient, measured at the maximum velocity point.
PGmid (Average Gradient) - The sum of the gradients measured every 2 seconds, divided by the number of measurements.

VTI

VTI (Velocity Time Integral) is calculated by the formula:

$$VTI = Vmid \times ET$$

SPECTRAL DOPPLER MEASUREMENTS

ET (Ejection Time) - The time from opening to closing the valve.

PHT

Pressure half-time (PHT) is the millisecond interval between the maximum gradient and the time point where the gradient is half the maximum initial value.

Ultrasound device will automatically do spectral Doppler measurements (Vmax, Vmid, PGmax, PGmid, VTI, PHT) when the user selects the appropriate spectrogram.

Using the Trans-mitral diastolic and LVOT flows spectrogram, the following parameters can be measured and calculated:

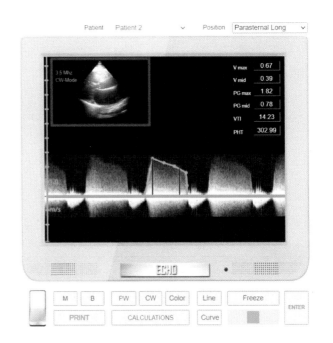

Spectral doppler measurements. V max, V mid, PG max, PG mid, VTI and PHT. Simulation By Echocardiography Online Simulator MyEchocardiography.com

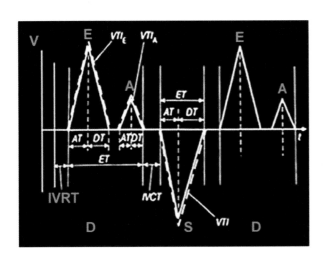

- **AT** (Acceleration Time) - The time from the opening of the mitral valve to the peak flow.
- **DT** (Deceleration Time) - the time from the Peak to Baseline.
- **ET** (Ejection Time) - The time from opening to closing the mitral valve.
- **Vmid** (Average Flow Velocity) - The sum of the flow velocities measured every 2 seconds, divided by the number of measurements.
- **VTI** (Velocity Time Integral) - *VTI = Vmid x ET*
- **Vmax** - Maximum flow velocity.
- **IVRT** - Isovolumetric relaxation time.
- **IVST** - Isovolumetric contraction time.

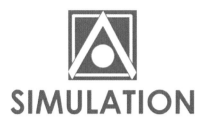

SIMULATION
SPECTRAL DOPPLER MEASUREMENTS
Echocardiography Online Simulator
MyEchocardiography.com

- Go to the link https://simulation.myechocardiography.com/

- Run Echocardiography Online Simulator using the **On/Off** Button

- Choose the patient from the list **<<Patient>>** Patient   Patient 1   ⌄

- Choose a position from the List **<<Positions>>** or Find a position with the 3D Transducer.

- Get Spectral Doppler on Display (PW or CW).

First way: We will get values for V max, PG max, and PHT

- Click the button **<<Line>>** Line   Put the first point on the maximum end of the spectrogram. Put another point in the place where velocity starts falling.

- Click the button **<<Enter>>**

Second way: we will get all values: V max, V mid, PG max, PG mid, VTI and PHT.

- Click the button **<<Curve>>** Curve   put points around spectrogram.

- Click the button **<<Enter>>**

- To change the patient, click the **On/Off** Button

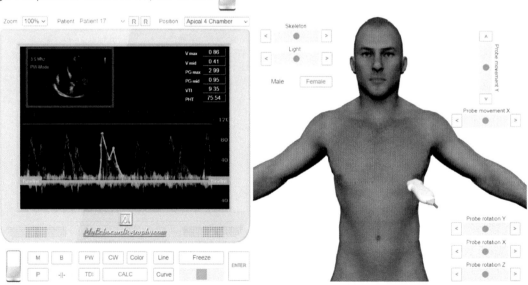

Apical 4-chamber view. PW Doppler. SPECTRAL DOPPLER MEASUREMENTS. Simulation By Echocardiography Online Simulator MyEchocardiography.com

https://youtu.be/iEWm-3bUXTU

SYSTOLIC AND DIASTOLIC FUNCTION OF THE LEFT VENTRICLE

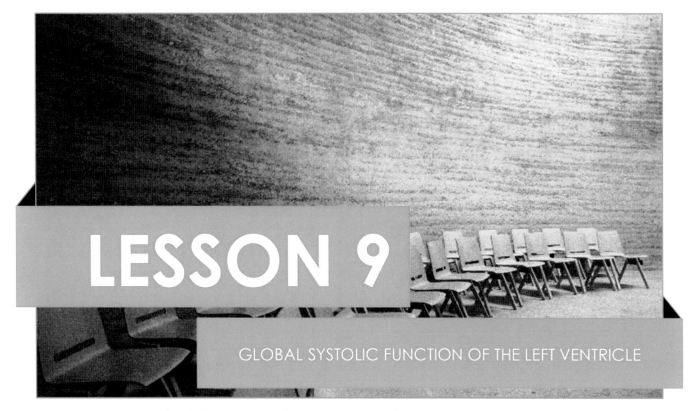

LESSON 9

GLOBAL SYSTOLIC FUNCTION OF THE LEFT VENTRICLE

There are various methods for assessing the global contractility of the left ventricle.

The following calculations are used:
- Ejection fraction.
- Fractional shortening.
- Stroke volume.
- Minute volume.
- Heart index.

Ejection Fraction

The Ejection Fraction (EF%) is the percentage ratio of the systolic volume of the left ventricle to the diastolic volume.

$$EF\% = \frac{LVEDV - LVESV}{LVEDV} \times 100$$

LVEDV - Left ventricular end-diastolic volume. LVESV - Left ventricular end-systolic volume.

The volume of the left ventricle can be measured using the Single plane or Biplane method.
If using the Single plane method, end-systolic and end-diastolic volume is better to measure in the Apical four-chamber position.
The Biplane method measures end-systolic and end-diastolic volume in two orthogonal positions (Apical four-chamber and Apical two-chamber view).

LESSON CONTENT

GLOBAL SYSTOLIC FUNCTION

- Ejection fraction.
- Fractional shortening.
- Stroke volume.
- Minute volume.
- Heart index.
- Body surface area (BSA)

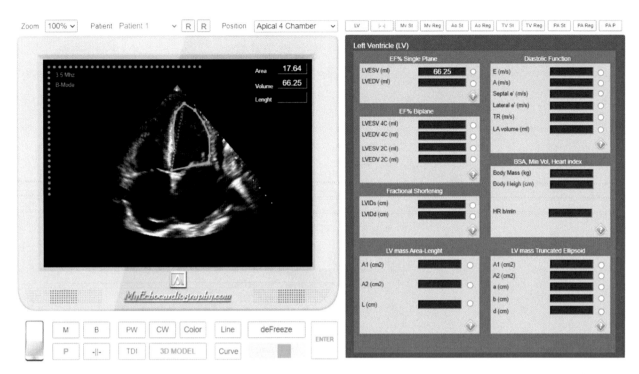

EF% calculation. Single Plane Method. Measurement of the end-systolic Volume. Simulation By Echocardiography Online Simulator MyEchocardiography.com

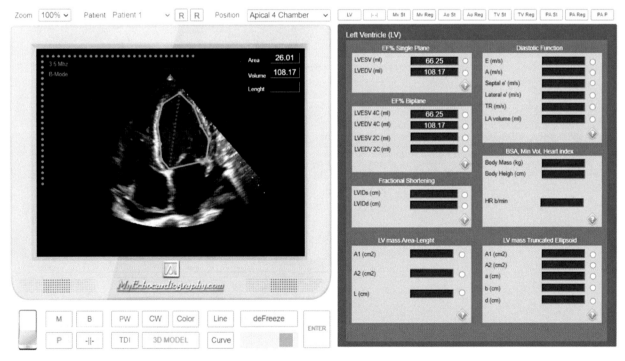

EF% calculation. Single Plane Method. Measurement of the end-diastolic Volume. Simulation By Echocardiography Online Simulator MyEchocardiography.com

LV GLOBAL SYSTOLIC FUNCTION

Stroke volume

Stroke volume is the blood pumped by the heart during one contraction.

$$SV = LVEDV - LVESV$$

Fractional shortening

The Fractional shortening (FS%) is the percentage ratio of the systolic Diameter of the left ventricle to the diastolic Diameter.

$$FS\% = \frac{LVEDD - LVESD}{LVEDD} \times 100$$

LVEDD - Left ventricular end-diastolic diameter. LVESD - Left ventricular end-systolic diameter.

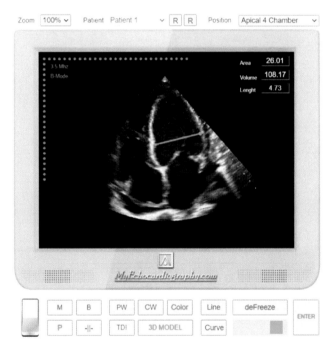

FS% calculation. Measurement of the end-diastolic Diameter. Simulation By Echocardiography Online Simulator MyEchocardiography.com

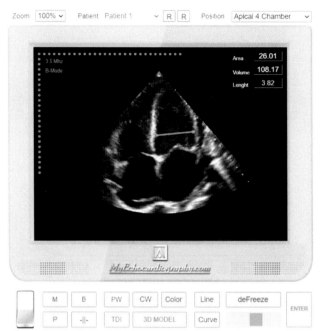

FS% calculation. Measurement of the end-systolic Diameter. Simulation By Echocardiography Online Simulator MyEchocardiography.com

Minute volume

Minute volume is the blood pumped by the heart in one minute.

$$CO = SV \times HR$$

SV-Stroke volume. HR-Heart rate.

Heart index

The Heart index is the ratio of the heart's minute volume to the body's surface area.

$$CI = \frac{CO}{BSA}$$

CO-Minute volume. BSA - Body surface area.

Body surface area (BSA)

The Du Bois formula can calculate body surface area:

$$BSA = M^{0.425} \times H^{0.725} \times 0.007184$$

M - Body weight (kg). H - Body Height (cm).

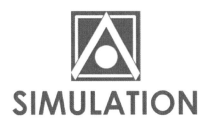

SIMULATION

LV EJECTION FRACTION, STROKE VOLUME, MINUTE VOLUME AND HEART INDEX

Echocardiography Online Simulator
MyEchocardiography.com

- Go to the link https://simulation.myechocardiography.com/
- Run Echocardiography Online Simulator using the **On/Off** Button
- Choose the patient from the list **<<Patient>>** Patient Patient 1 ⌄

Singe-Plane Method:

- Choose 4 chamber position from the List **<<Positions>>** or find 4 chamber position with **3D Transducer**
- Click the button **<<Freeze>>** to freeze image. Using **Slider** find LV End - Systolic frame.
- Click Button **<<Calculations>>** Click Tab **<<LV>>** Click Radio Button **<<LVESV (ml)>>** in the Panel "EF% Single Plane".
- Measure LV Volume *(see the lesson 7)*
- Click the button **<<Enter>>**
- Using **Slider** find LV End-Diastolic frame.
- Click Radio Button **<<LVEDV D (ml)>>** in the Panel "EF% Single Plane".
- Measure LV Volume (see the lesson 7)
- For the Calculation of the **Minute volume** and **Heart index** enter the Body Mass (kg), Body Heigh (cm) and Heart rate (b/min) in the Tab "BSA, Min Vol, Heart index".
- Click the button **<<Enter>>**
- Click the button << R >> to see the results.

Bi-Plane Method:

- Choose 4 chamber position from the List **<<Positions>>** or find 4 chamber position with **3D Transducer**
- Click the button **<<Freeze>>** to freeze image. Using **Slider** find LV End - Systolic frame.
- Click Button **<<Calculations>>** Click Tab **<<LV>>** Click Radio Button **<<LVESV $C (ml)>>** in the Panel "EF% Biplane".
- Measure LV Volume *(see the lesson 7)*
- Click the button **<<Enter>>**

- Using **Slider** find LV End-Diastolic frame.
- Click Radio Button **<<LVEDV 4C (ml)>>** in the Panel "EF% Biplane".
- Measure LV Volume (see the lesson 7)
- Click the button **<<Enter>>**
- Choose 2 chamber position from the List **<<Positions>>** or find 2 chamber position with **3D Transducer**
- Click the button **<<Freeze>>** to freeze image. Using **Slider** find LV End - Systolic frame.
- Click Radio Button **<<LVESV 2C (ml)>>** in the Panel "EF% Biplane".
- Measure LV Volume (see the lesson 7)
- Click the button **<<Enter>>**
- Using **Slider** find LV End-Diastolic frame.
- Click Radio Button **<<LVEDV 2C (ml)>>** in the Panel "EF% Biplane"
- Measure LV Volume (see the lesson 7)
- For the Calculation of the **Minute volume** and **Heart index** enter the Body Mass (kg), Body Heigh (cm) and Heart rate (b/min) in the Tab "BSA, Min Vol, Heart index".
- Click the button **<<Enter>>**
- Click the button << **R** >> to see the results.
- To change the patient, click the **On/Off** Button

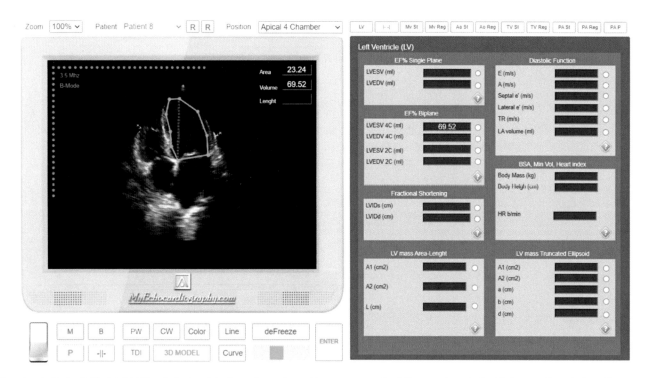

EF% calculation. Biplane Method. Apical 4 chamber view. Measurement of the end-systolic Volume. Simulation By Echocardiography Online Simulator MyEchocardiography.com

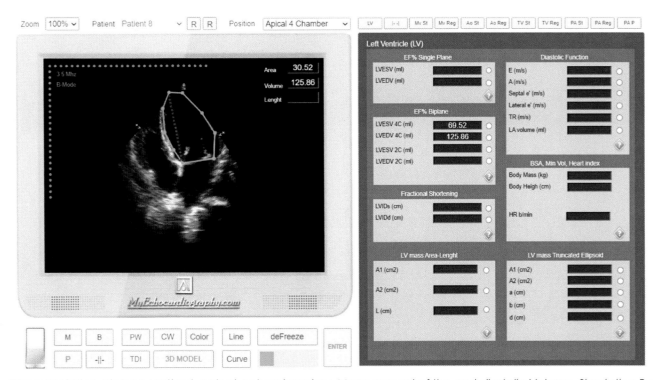

EF% calculation. Biplane Method. Apical 4 chamber view. Measurement of the end-diastolic Volume. Simulation By Echocardiography Online Simulator MyEchocardiography.com

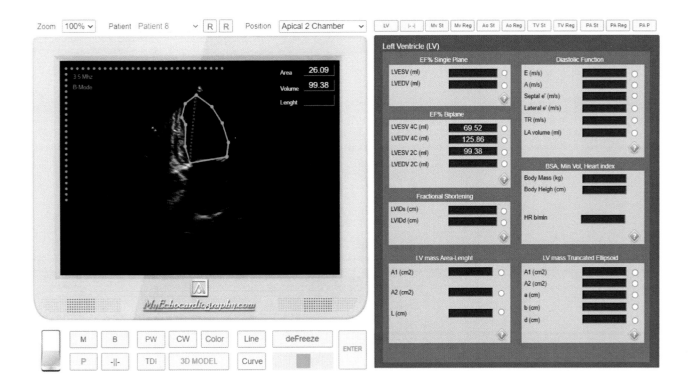

EF% calculation. Biplane Method. Apical 2 chamber view. Measurement of the end-systolic Volume. Simulation By Echocardiography Online Simulator MyEchocardiography.com

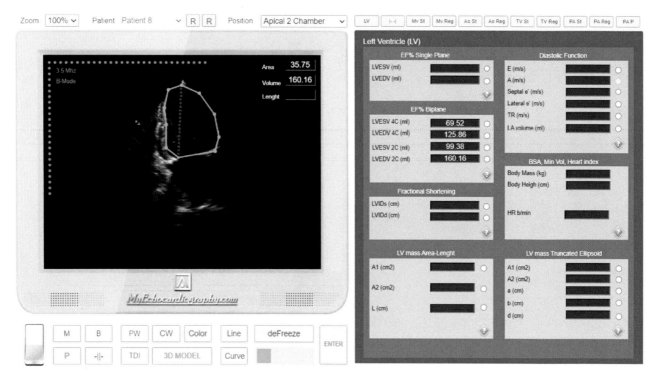

EF% calculation. Biplane Method. Apical 2 chamber view. Measurement of the end-diastolic Volume. Simulation By Echocardiography Online Simulator MyEchocardiography.com

https://www.youtube.com/watch?v=XhjG669HvYI&t=70s

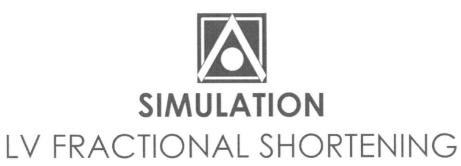

SIMULATION
LV FRACTIONAL SHORTENING
Echocardiography Online Simulator
MyEchocardiography.com

- Go to the link https://simulation.myechocardiography.com/

- Run Echocardiography Online Simulator using the **On/Off** Button

- Choose the patient from the list **<<Patient>>** Patient   Patient 1   ⌄

- Choose 4 chamber position from the List **<<Positions>>** or find 4 chamber position with **3D Transducer**

- Click the button **<<Freeze>>** to freeze image. Using **Slider** find LV End - Systolic frame.

- Click Button **<<Calculations>>** Click Tab **<<LV>>** Click Radio Button **<< LVIDs (cm)>>** in the Panel "Fractional Shortening".

- Measure LV end-systolic internal diameter *(see the lesson 6)*

- Click the button **<<Enter>>**

- Click Radio Button **<< LVIDd (cm)>>** in the Panel "Fractional Shortening".

- Using **Slider** find LV End-diastolic frame.

- Measure LV end-diastolic internal diameter (see the lesson 6)

- Click the button **<<Enter>>**

- Click the button << R >> to see the results.

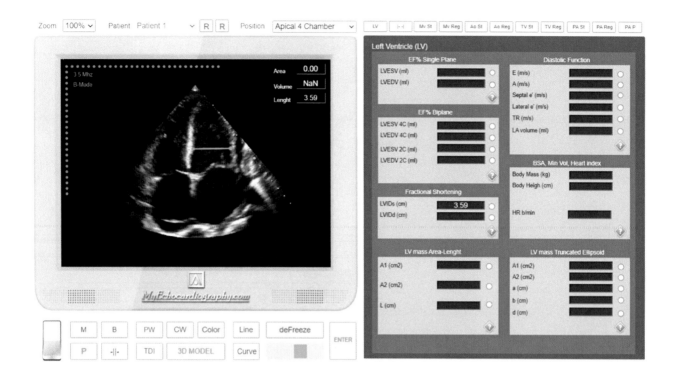

FS% calculation. Apical 4 chamber view. Measurement of the end-systolic Diameter. Simulation By Echocardiography Online Simulator MyEchocardiography.com

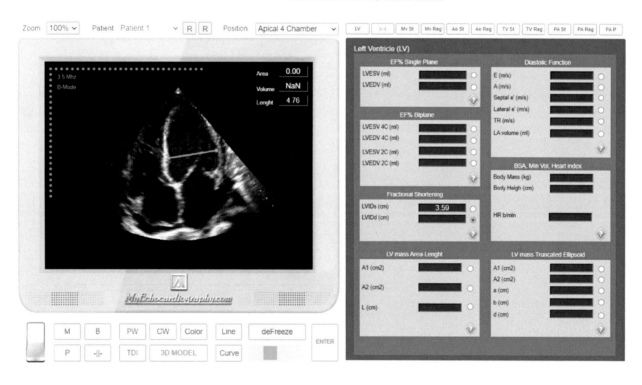

FS% calculation. Apical 4 chamber view. Measurement of the end-diastolic Diameter. Simulation By Echocardiography Online Simulator MyEchocardiography.com

https://www.youtube.com/watch?v=6bFnQ3h7fbQ

LV Mass

The American Society of Echocardiography (ASE) recommends the use of the following two methods for left ventricular mass assessment:

- The "Area-length" method.
- The "Truncated ellipsoid" method.

Method "Area-lenght"

$$LV_{mass} = 1.05\left[\frac{5}{6}A_1(L+t)\right] - \left[\frac{5}{6}A_2L\right]$$

$$t = \sqrt{A_1/\pi} - \sqrt{A_2/\pi}$$

A1 - Epicardial area (cm2). A2 - Endocardial area (cm2). L - Long axis of the left ventricle (cm). t - Mean wall thickness (cm).

In the Left parasternal position, at the level of papillary muscles, contours are drawn around the endocardium and epicardium (at the end of diastole). When tracing the endocardium, ignore the papillary muscles. Ultrasound devices will automatically calculate the area (A1, A2). The myocardial area is obtained by subtracting the endocardial area from the epicardial.

The long axis of the left ventricle is measured in the Apical four-chamber or two-chamber position at the end of the diastole.

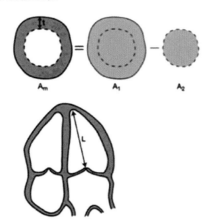

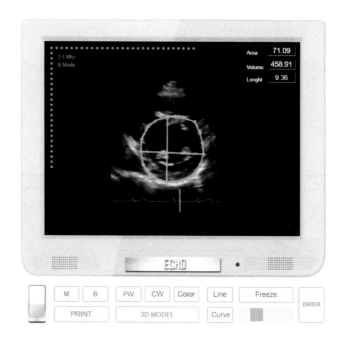

LV mass. Left parasternal view, at the level of the papillary muscles. Measurement of the Epicardial area (A1). Simulation By Echocardiography Online Simulator MyEchocardiography.com

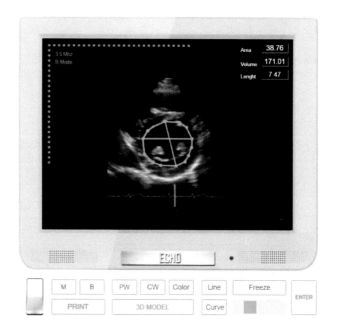

LV mass. Left parasternal view, at the level of the papillary muscles. Measurement of the Endocardial area (A2). Simulation By Echocardiography Online Simulator MyEchocardiography.com

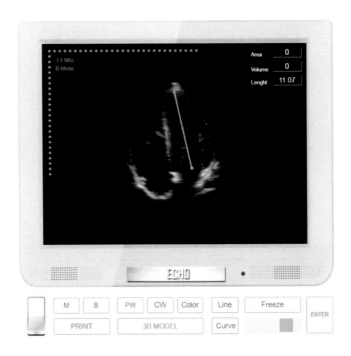

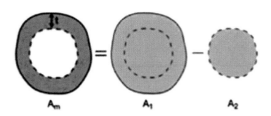

In the Left parasternal position, at the level of papillary muscles, contours are drawn around the endocardium and epicardium (at the end of diastole). When tracing the endocardium, ignore the papillary muscles.

Ultrasound devices will automatically calculate the area (A1, A2). The myocardial area is obtained by subtracting the endocardial area from the epicardial.

Then the left ventricle is presented as a "truncated ellipsoid." The long axis is divided into two parts at the level of the short axis of the left ventricle. Both parts (a, d) and the radius of the short axis (b) are measured.

Measurements must be done in the Apical four-chamber or two-chamber position at the end of the diastole.

LV mass. Method "Area-Lenght". Apical 4 chamber view. Measurement of the LV Long axis (L). Simulation By Echocardiography Online Simulator *MyEchocardiography.com*

Method "Truncated ellipsoid"

$$LV_{mass} = 1.05\pi (b+t)^2 \left[\frac{2}{3}(a+t) + d - \frac{d^3}{3(a+t)^2} \right] -$$

$$b^2 \left[\frac{2}{3}a + d - \frac{d^3}{3a^2} \right]$$

$$t = \sqrt{A_1/\pi} - \sqrt{A_2/\pi}$$

$$b = \sqrt{A_2/\pi}$$

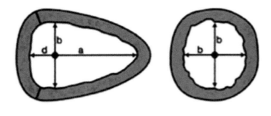

A1 - Epicardial area (cm2). A2 - Endocardial area (cm2). t - Mean wall thickness (cm). a - Long semi-axis of the left ventricle (cm). d - short semi-axis of the left ventricle (cm). b - Short axis radius (cm).

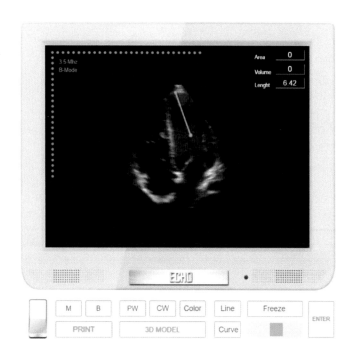

LV mass. Method "Truncated Ellipsoid". Apical 4 chamber view. Measurement of the Long semi-axis of the left ventricle (a).Simulation By Echocardiography Online Simulator MyEchocardiography.com

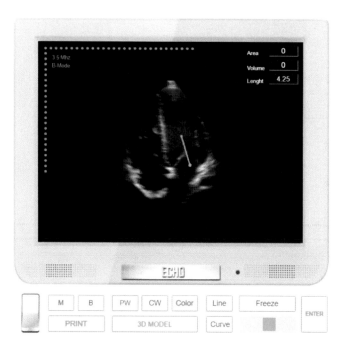

LV mass. Method "Truncated Ellipsoid". Apical 4 chamber view. Measurement of the short semi-axis of the left ventricle (d). Simulation By Echocardiography Online Simulator MyEchocardiography.com

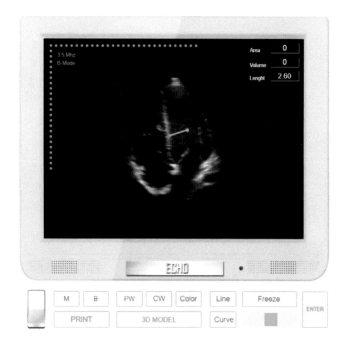

LV mass. Method "Truncated Ellipsoid". Apical 4 chamber view. Measurement of the short axis radius (b). Simulation By Echocardiography Online Simulator MyEchocardiography.com

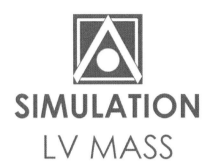

SIMULATION
LV MASS
Echocardiography Online Simulator
MyEchocardiography.com

- Go to the link https://simulation.myechocardiography.com/
- Run Echocardiography Online Simulator using the **On/Off** Button
- Choose the patient from the list **<<Patient>>** Patient Patient 1 ⌄

Method Area-Lenght:

- Choose Choose Parasternal Short PM (Left Parasternal View, Short axis of LV at the level of Papillary Muscles) From the List **<<Positions>>** or find the position with **3D Transducer**
- Click the button **<<Freeze>>** to freeze image. Using **Slider** find LV End - diastolic frame.
- Click Button **<<Calculations>>** Click Tab **<<LV>>** Click Radio Button **<<A1>>** in the Panel "LV mass Area-Lenght".
- Click the button **<<Curve>>** place points around epicardium and Click the button **<<Enter>>**
- Click Radio Button **<<A2>>** Click the button **<<Curve>>** place points around endocardium (ignore papillary muscles) and Click the button **<<Enter>>**
- Choose 4 chamber position from the List **<<Positions>>** or find 4 chamber position with **3D Transducer**
- Click the button **<<Freeze>>** to freeze image. Using **Slider** find LV End-diastolic frame.
- Click the Radio Button **<<L (cm)>>**
- Measure the long axis of the Left Ventricle.
- Click the button **<<Enter>>**
- Click the button << R >> to see the results.
- To change the patient, click the **On/Off** Button

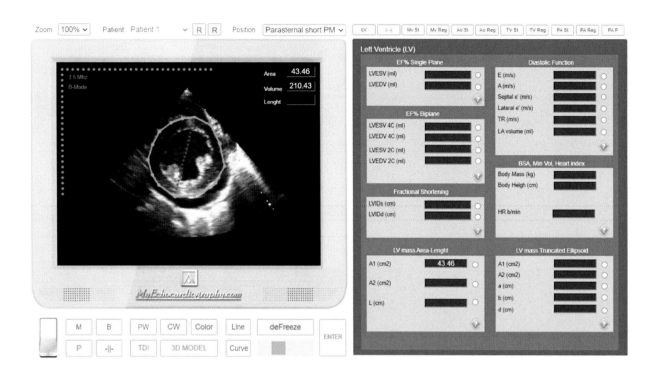

LV mass. Left parasternal view, at the level of the papillary muscles. Measurement of the Epicardial area (A1). Simulation By Echocardiography Online Simulator *MyEchocardiography.com*

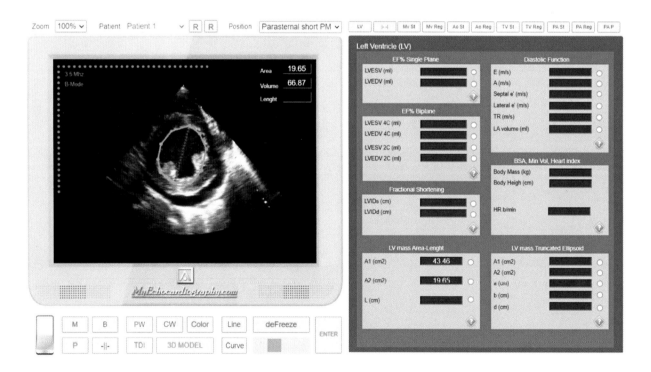

LV mass. Left parasternal view, at the level of the papillary muscles. Measurement of the Endocardial area (A2). Simulation By Echocardiography Online Simulator *MyEchocardiography.com*

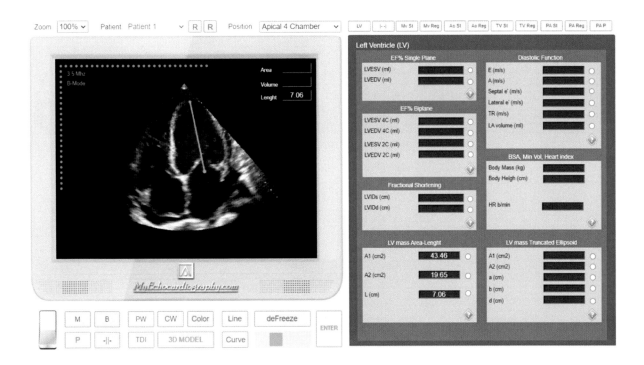

LV mass. Method "Area-Lenght". Apical 4 chamber view. Measurement of the LV Long axis (L). Simulation By Echocardiography Online Simulator MyEchocardiography.com

https://www.youtube.com/watch?v=h8qhWlkPuPM

Truncated Ellipsoid Method:

- Choose Choose Parasternal Short PM (Left Parasternal View, Short axis of LV at the level of Papillary Muscles) From the List **<<Positions>>** or <u>find the position with</u> **3D Transducer**
- Click the button **<<Freeze>>** to freeze image. Using **Slider** find LV End - diastolic frame.
- Click Button **<<Calculations>>** Click Tab **<<LV>>** Click Radio Button **<<A1>>** in the Panel "LV mass Area-Lenght".
- Click the button **<<Curve>>** place points around epicardium and Click the button **<<Enter>>**
- Click Radio Button **<<A2>>** Click the button **<<Curve>>** place points around endocardium (ignore papillary muscles) and Click the button **<<Enter>>**
- Choose 4 chamber position from the List **<<Positions>>** or <u>find the position with</u> **3D Transducer**
- Click the button **<<Freeze>>** to freeze image. Using **Slider** find LV End-diastolic frame.
- Click Radio Button **<<a>>** and measure distance from the minor axis to the endocardium
- Click the button **<<Enter>>**
- Click Radio Button **<<b>>** and measure the distance from the minor axis to the endocardium
- Measure the LV minor radius.
- Click the button **<<Enter>>**
- Click Radio Button **<<d>>** and measure the distance from the minor axis to the mitral valve plane.
- Click the button **<<Enter>>**
- Click the button << R >> to see the results.
- To change the patient, click the **On/Off** Button

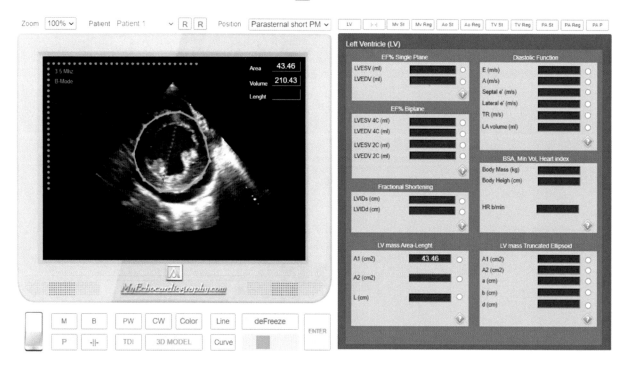

LV mass. Left parasternal view, at the level of the papillary muscles. Measurement of the Epicardial area (A1). Simulation By Echocardiography Online Simulator MyEchocardiography.com

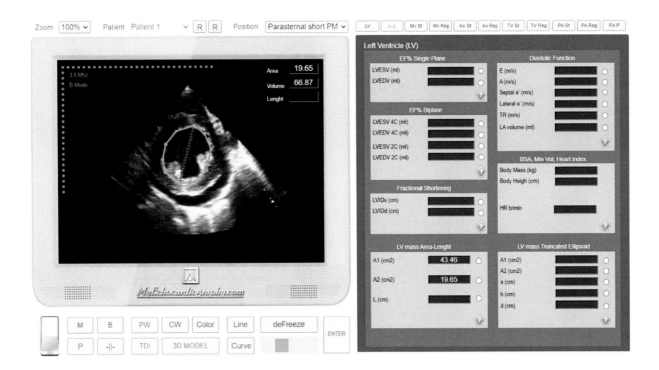

LV mass. Left parasternal view, at the level of the papillary muscles. Measurement of the Endocardial area (A2). Simulation By Echocardiography Online Simulator MyEchocardiography.com

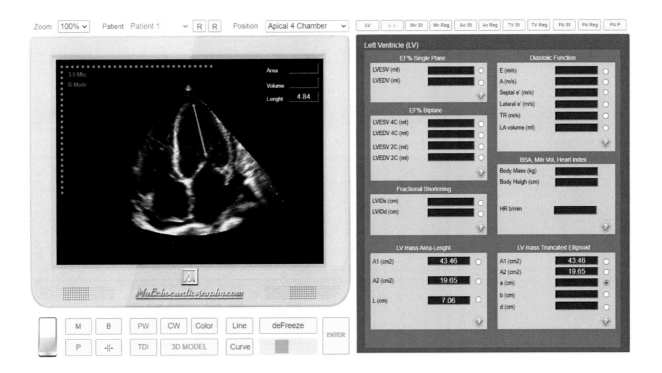

LV mass. Method "Truncated Ellipsoid". Apical 4 chamber view. Measurement of the Long semi-axis of the left ventricle (a).Simulation By Echocardiography Online Simulator MyEchocardiography.com

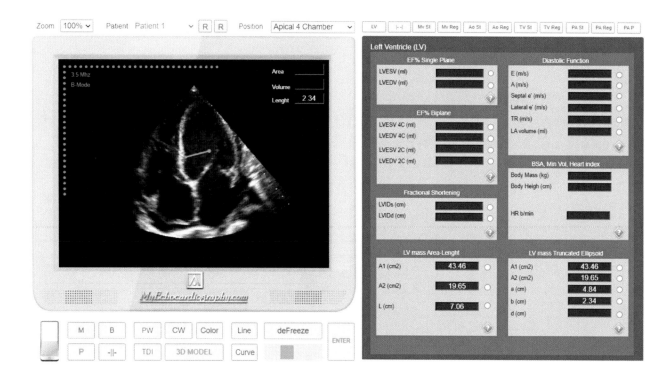

LV mass. Method "Truncated Ellipsoid". Apical 4 chamber view. Measurement of the short axis radius (b). Simulation By Echocardiography Online Simulator MyEchocardiography.com

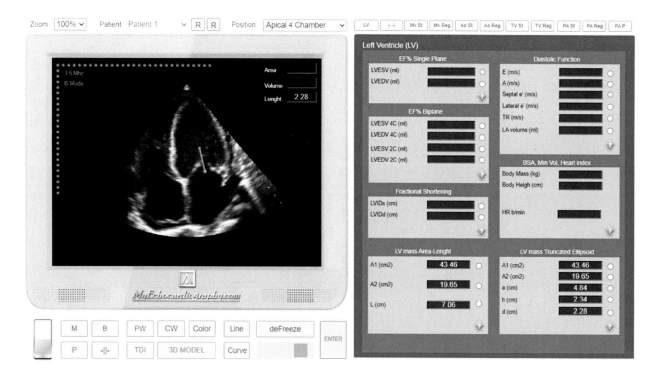

LV mass. Method "Truncated Ellipsoid". Apical 4 chamber view. Measurement of the short semi-axis of the left ventricle (d). Simulation By Echocardiography Online Simulator MyEchocardiography.com

https://www.youtube.com/watch?v=h8qhWlkPuPM

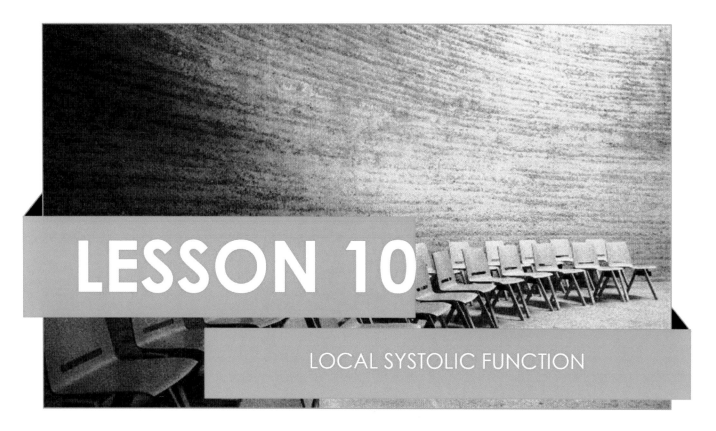

LESSON 10

LOCAL SYSTOLIC FUNCTION

The American Association of Echocardiography (ASE) recommends using a 16-segment model to assess regional myocardial contractility based on the following:

- Anatomical logic.
- Easy identification of each segment with anatomical boundaries.
- The connection of each segment to the blood supply from a particular coronary artery.

This model divides the myocardium into three levels and 16 segments. When dividing into levels, the papillary muscles are considered the anatomical border.

- Basal level (Basal) - from the mitral valve's fibrous ring to the papillary muscles' end.
- Middle level (Mid) - from the end of the papillary muscles to its beginning.
- Apical level - from the beginning of the papillary muscles to the top of the heart.

The basal and middle levels are divided into six equal segments, and the apical level is divided into four segments.

It is possible to classify each segment according to the blood supply of 3 coronary arteries (We should consider differences between the individuals in the coronary blood supply).

LOCAL SYSTOLIC FUNCTION

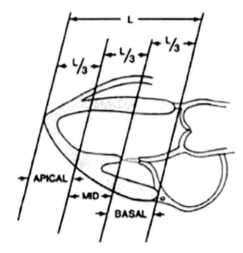

Division of the left ventricle into basal, middle, and apical levels. Left parasternal position, long axis.

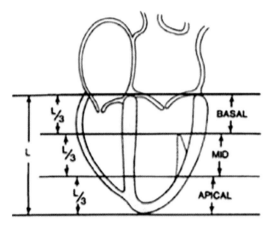

Division of the left ventricle into basal, middle, and apical levels. Apical 4 chamber view.

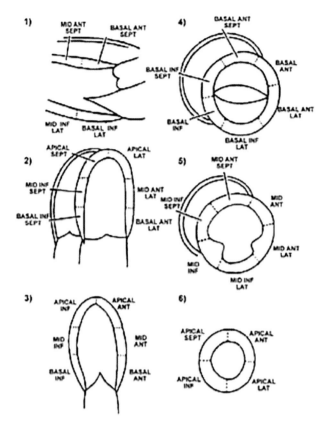

Division of myocardium into 16 segments for two-dimensional echocardiography. 1. Left parasternal view, long axis. 2. Apical four-chamber view. 3. Apical two-chamber view. 4. Left parasternal view, short axis, at the level of the mitral valve. 5. Left parasternal view, short axis, at the level of the papillary muscles. 6. Apex.

LOCAL SYSTOLIC FUNCTION

The regional contractility assessment system is based on the assessment of each segment.

Recommended quantitative criteria for the assessment of regional contractility:

- Normal contractility - systolic increase in ventricular wall thickness by more than 50% (1 point).

- Hypokinesia - systolic increase in ventricular wall thickness less than 40% (2 points).

- Akinesia - systolic increase in ventricular wall thickness of less than 10% (3 points).

- Dyskinesia - depression on the opposite side of the wall during systole and its thinning (4 points).

- Aneurysm - concavation on the opposite side of the wall during systole, dilatation, systolic thinning, and diastolic deformation remains during the diastole phase (5 points).

The following formula calculates the regional contractility index:

$$I = \frac{\sum S}{n}$$

I - regional compressibility index. Counter - sum of points of evaluated segments. Denominator - the number of evaluated segments.

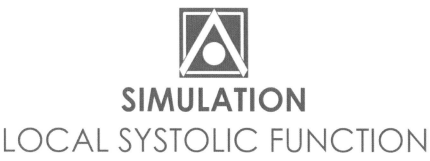

SIMULATION
LOCAL SYSTOLIC FUNCTION
Echocardiography Online Simulator
MyEchocardiography.com

- Go to the link https://simulation.myechocardiography.com/

- Run Echocardiography Online Simulator using the **On/Off** Button

- Choose the patient from the list **<<Patient>>**

- Choose one of the positions in which local systolic function can be assessed **<<Parasternal Long>>**,
  <<Parasternal Short MV>>, **<<Parasternal Short PM>>**, **<<Parasternal Short Apex>>**, **<<Apical 4 Chamber>>**.
  <<Apical 2 Chamber>> or find the position with **3D Transducer**

- Click Button **<<Calculations>>** Click Tab **<<|--|>>**

- Examine Each segment of the heart and choose the condition from the specific Lists

- Click the button **<< R >>** to see the results.

- To change the patient, click the **On/Off** Button

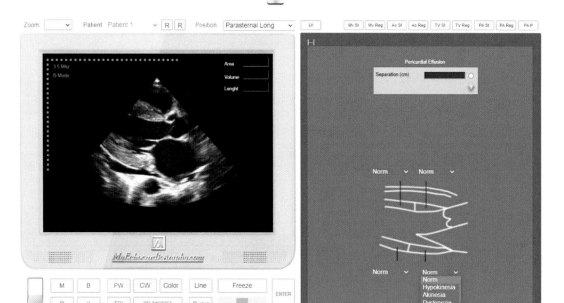

*Left Parasternal View, Short axis. Assessment of the LV Local systolic function. Simulation By
Echocardiography Online Simulator MyEchocardiography.com*

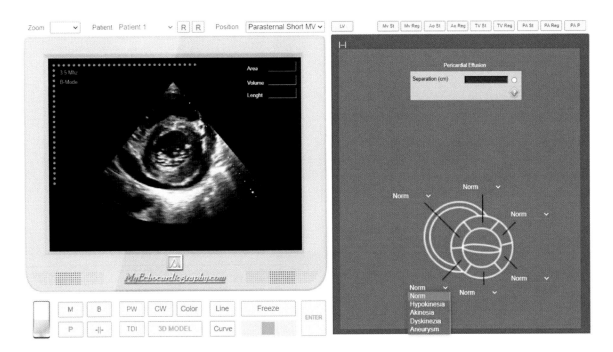

Left Parasternal View, Short axis at the level of the mitral valve. Assessment of the LV Local systolic function.
Simulation By Echocardiography Online Simulator MyEchocardiography.com

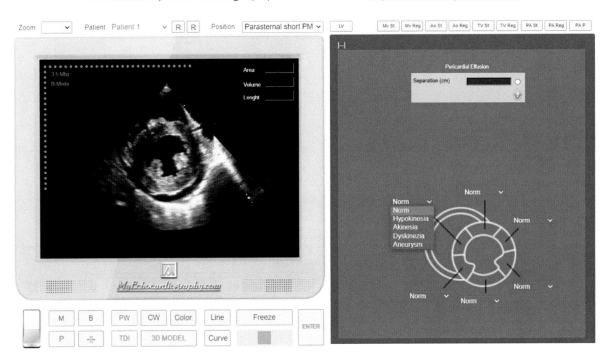

Left Parasternal View, Short axis at the level of the Papillary Muscles. Assessment of the LV Local systolic function.
Simulation By Echocardiography Online Simulator MyEchocardiography.com

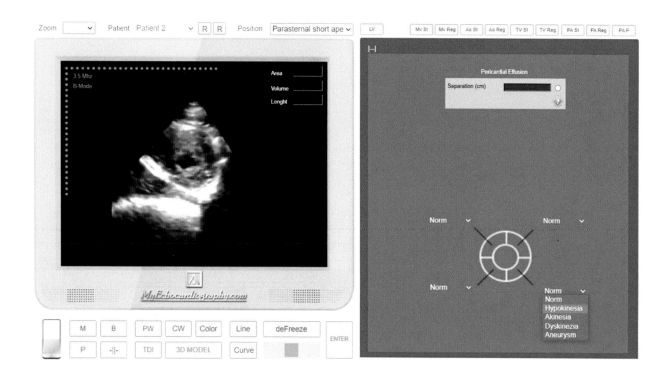

Left Parasternal View, Short axis at the level of the Heart Apex. Assessment of the LV Local systolic function. Simulation By Echocardiography Online Simulator MyEchocardiography.com

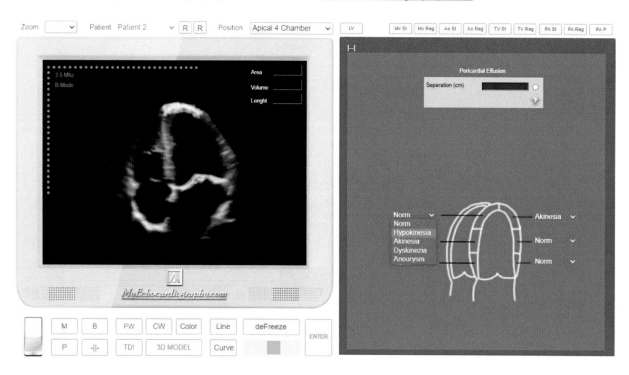

Apical Four Chamber View, Short axis at the level of the Heart Apex. Assessment of the LV Local systolic function. Simulation By Echocardiography Online Simulator MyEchocardiography.com

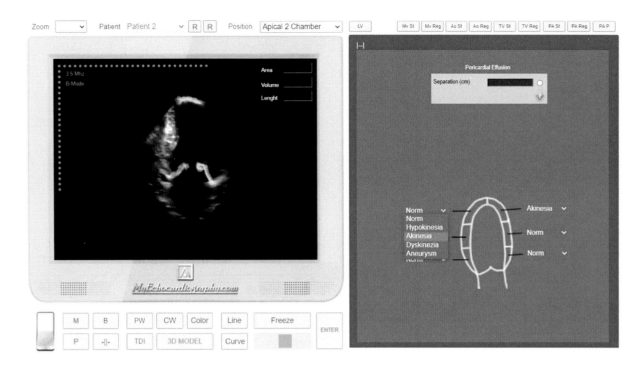

Apical Two Chamber View, Short axis at the level of the Heart Apex. Assessment of the LV Local systolic function.
Simulation By Echocardiography Online Simulator MyEchocardiography.com

https://youtu.be/P9qsiotnlqg

LESSON 11

LEFT VENTRICULAR DIASTOLIC FUNCTION

According to the guidelines from the American Society of Echocardiography (ASE), There are two algorithms for evaluating the left ventricular diastolic function.
First - for the patients with the normal Left Ventricular Ejection Fraction (EF%). second - for the patients with depressed EF% and patients with myocardial disease and normal EF (after consideration of clinical and other 2D data).

LESSON CONTENT

LV Diastolic Function

- Assessment in patient with Normal EF%.
- Assessment in patient with depressed EF% and patients with myocardial disease.
- Simulation By Echocardiography Online Simulator MyEchocardiography.com

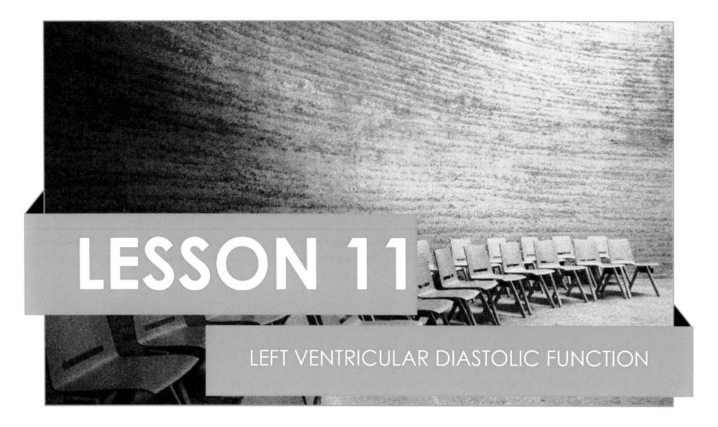

In patients with normal LV EF

1-Average E/e' > 14
2-Septal e' velocity < 7 cm/s or Lateral e' velocity <10 cm/s
3-TR velocity > 2.8 m/s
4-LA volume index >34ml/m²

| <50% positive | 50% positive | >50% positive |

| Normal Diastolic function | Indeterminate | Diastolic Dysfunction |

Algorithm for diagnosis of LV diastolic dysfunction in subjects with normal LV EF%.

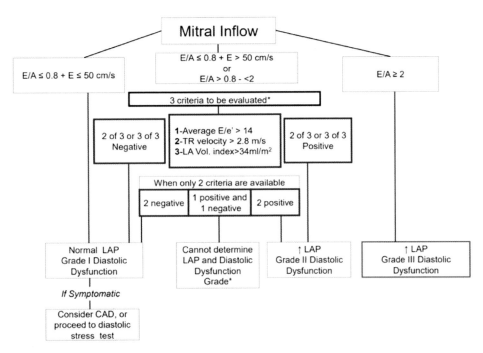

Algorithm for estimation of LV filling pressures and grading LV diastolic function in patients with depressed EF% and patients with myocardial disease and normal EF% (after consideration of clinical and other 2D data).

If the LV EF% is normal (and the patient has no myocardial disease), the first algorithm has to be used. In this case, we have to measure five parameters.	If the LV EF% is depressed or EF% is normal, but the patient has myocardial disease, the second algorithm must be used. In this case, we have to measure six parameters.
<ul><li>**E** - Maximal velocity of the Transmitral Diastolic Flow (peak E, spectral Doppler).</li><li>**Septal e'** - Septal e' velocity on Tissue Doppler.</li><li>**Lateral e'** - Lateral e' velocity on Tissue Doppler.</li><li>**TR velocity** - Tricuspid regurgitation velocity.</li><li>**LA Volume index** - Left Atrial Volume index (for calculation, we need LA volume and Body Surface Area - BSA).</li></ul>	<ul><li>**E** - Maximal velocity of the Early Diastolic Filling (peak E, spectral Doppler).</li><li>**A** - Maximal velocity of the Late Diastolic Filling (peak A, spectral Doppler).</li><li>**Septal e'** - Septal e' velocity on Tissue Doppler.</li><li>**Lateral e'** - Lateral e' velocity on Tissue Doppler.</li><li>**TR velocity** - Tricuspid regurgitation velocity.</li><li>**LA Volume index** - Left Atrial Volume index (for calculation, we need LA volume and Body Surface Area - BSA).</li></ul>

Using Echocardiography Online Simulator MyEchocardiography.com users can simulate all stages of assessment of the LV Diastolic Function

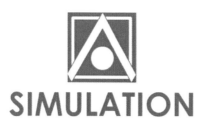

SIMULATION
LEFT VENTRICULAR DIASTOLIC FUNCTION

Echocardiography Online Simulator
MyEchocardiography.com

- Go to the link https://simulation.myechocardiography.com/
- Run Echocardiography Online Simulator using the **On/Off** Button

From the beginning, the user needs to Calculate LV Ejection Fraction (EF%). Calculations are different in patients with normal EF% than those with depressed EF%.

After Calculating EF% user can start the Evaluation of the Left Ventricular Diastolic Function:

- From the List **<<Patients>>** Choose Patient 9 (User can Choose other patients as well).
- Choose **4 chamber** position from the List **<<Positions>>** or find the position with **3D Transducer**
- Click Button **<<Calculations>>** Click Tab **<<LV>>** Find Panel **"Diastolic Function"** and Click Radio Button **<<E m/s >>**
- Click the button **<<PW>>** to start Pulse Wave doppler examination. Place Control Volume Beetwen Mitral Valve Leaflets and Click.
- For Mitral Inflow "E" point velocity measurement, click the button **<<Line>>**. Put first point on the maximum point of the spectrogram. Put another point on baseline.
- Click the button <<Enter>>

* If EF% is depressed, we need to Measure "A" point Velocity as well.

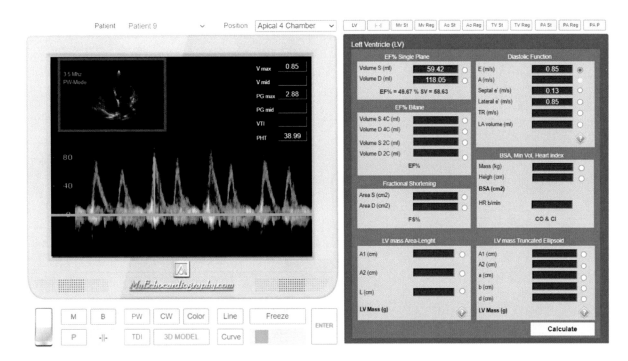

Measurement of the Maximal velocity of trans mitral diastolic flow. Simulation By Echocardiography Online Simulator MyEchocardiography.com

- In the Tab **<<LV>>** Find Panel **"Diastolic Function"** and Click Radio Button **<<Septal e' m/s >>**
- Click The button **<<2D>>** to move to the 2D examination.
- Click the button **<<TDI>>** to start the Tissue Doppler examination. Place Control Volume in the septal side of the mitral annulus and **Click**.

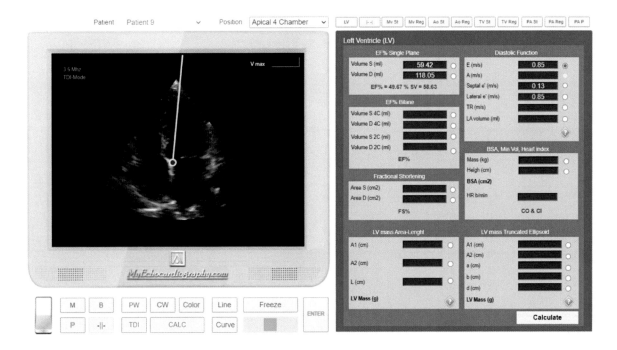

Apical 4 chamber view. Control Volume position for the Septal TDI. Simulation By Echocardiography Online Simulator MyEchocardiography.com

- Click the button **<<Line>>** put the first point on the maximum point of the e' wave. Put another point on Baseline.
- Click the button **<<Enter>>**

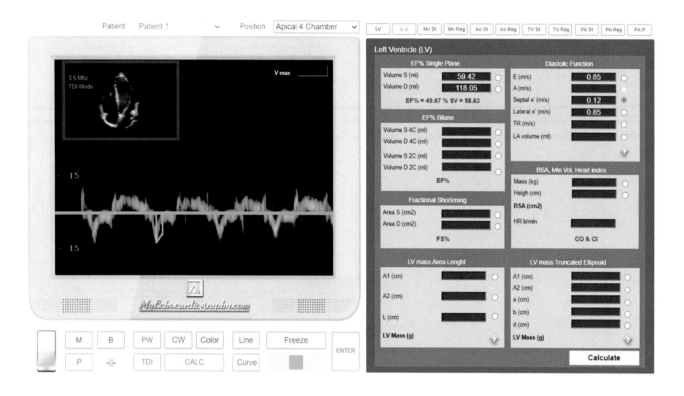

Tissue Doppler (TDI). Measuremen of Septal e' (V max). Simulation By Echocardiography Online Simulator MyEchocardiography.com

- In the Tab **<<LV>>** Find Panel **"Diastolic Function"** and Click Radio Button **<<Septal e' m/s >>**
- Click the **<<2D>>** button to move to the 2D examination.
- Click the **<<TDI>>** button to start the Tissue Doppler examination. Place Control Volume on the lateral side of the mitral annulus and **Click**.

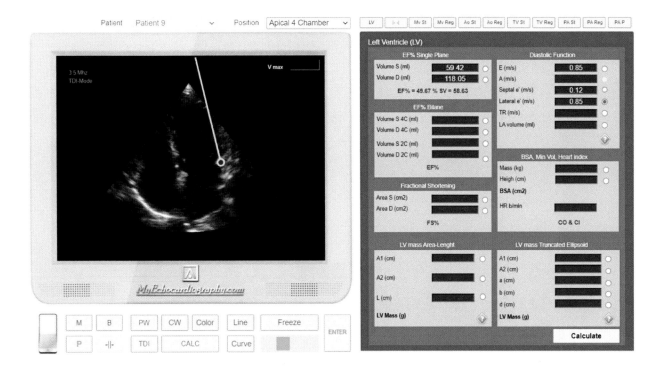

Apical 4 chamber view. Control Volume position for the Lateral TDI. Simulation By Echocardiography Online Simulator MyEchocardiography.com

- Click the button **<<Line>>**. Put first point on the maximum point of the e' wave. Put another point on Baseline.
- Click the button **<<Enter>>**

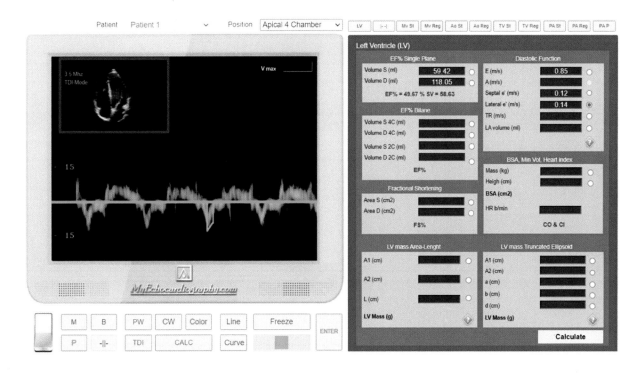

Tissue Doppler (TDI). Measuremen of the Lateral e' (V max). Simulation By Echocardiography Online Simulator MyEchocardiography.com

- Click the **<<PW>>** button to start the Pulse Wave Doppler examination. Place Control Volume between Tricuspid Valve Leaflets and **Click**.
- Click the button **<<Curve>>**. Put points around the tricuspid regurgitation jet.
- Click the button **<<Enter>>**

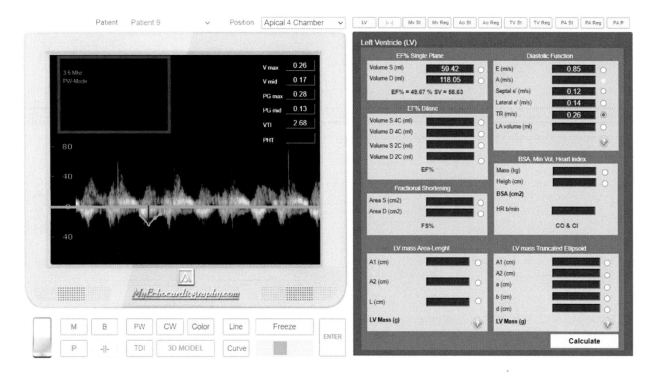

Measurement of the Tricuspid regurgitation velosity. Simulation By Echocardiography Online Simulator MyEchocardiography.com

- In the Tab **<<LV>>**, Find Panel **"Diastolic Function"** and Click Radio Button **<<LA Volume (ml) >>**
- Click The button **<<2D>>** to move to the 2D examination.
- Click the button **<<Freeze>>** to freeze the image. Using **Slider,** find the best position for LA Volume measurement.
- Click the button **<<Curve>>** and trace around the inner side of the LA endocardium.
- Click the button **<<Enter>>**

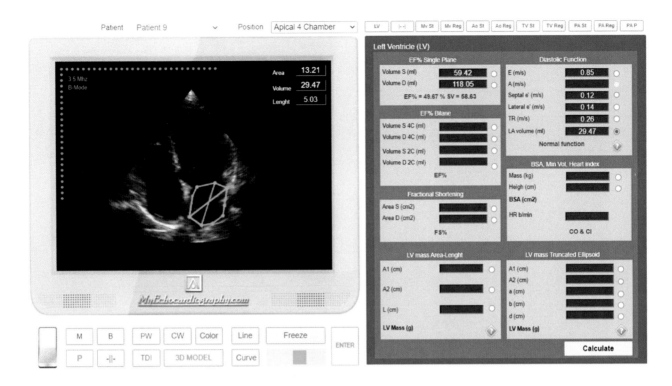

Left Atrium (LA) Volume measurement. Simulation By Echocardiography Online Simulator <u>MyEchocardiography.com</u>

<u>https://www.youtube.com/watch?v=xJBbc8kR-RI</u>

VALVULAR

PATHOLOGIES

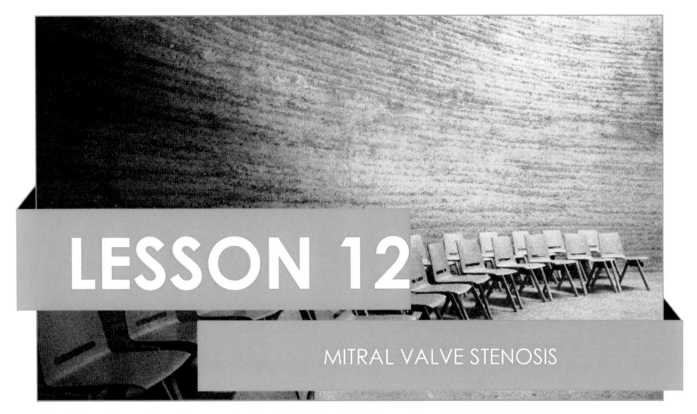

LESSON 12

Mitral stenosis can be diagnosed using M-Mode, B-Mode, and spectral Doppler.

Mitral stenosis

- Diagnosis of mitral stenosis.
- Mitral Valve Area by Tracing.
- Mitral Valve Area by PHT.
- Mitral Valve Area (CONTINUITY EQUATION).
- Degree of Mitral Stenosis by Mean Pressure Gradient.

One-Dimensional Echocardiography (M-Mode)

- Decrease in the rate of diastolic closure of the anterior leaflet of the mitral valve.
- Unilateral movement of the mitral valve anterior and posterior leaflets.

Due to the high pressure in the left atrium during diastole, the valve leaflets remain open and, unlike the norm, do not close after the left ventricle early rapid filling.
The curve of the mitral valve movement has a ⊓-shaped form instead of an M-shaped one.

The unilateral movement of the anterior and posterior leaflets of the mitral valve can be seen due to the fusion of the leaflets. (Normally, the leaflets move in different directions).

MITRAL STENOSIS

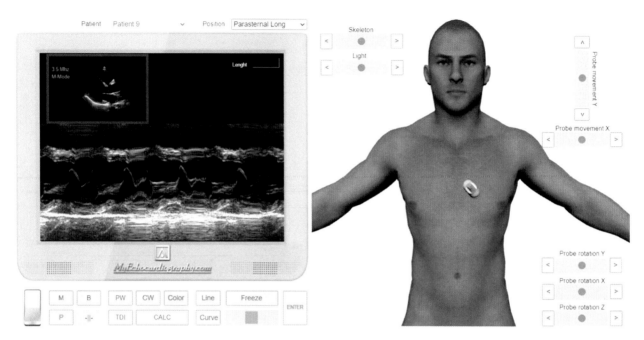

Left parasternal view, the lond axis of the heart. One dimensional Echocardiography (m-mode). Normal Mitral Valve. Simulation By Echocardiography Online Simulator MyEchocardiography.com

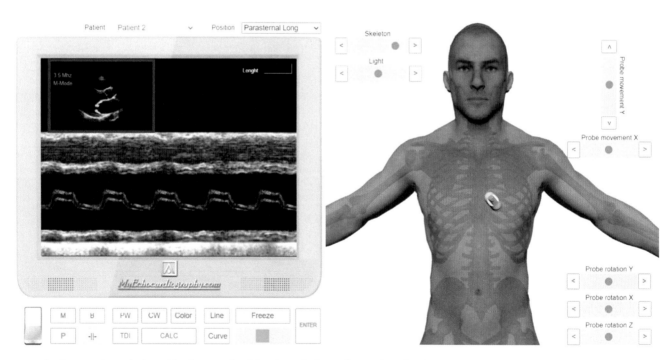

Left parasternal view, the long axis of the heart. One-dimensional Echocardiography (m-mode). Mitral Stenosis. Decrease in the rate of diastolic closure of the anterior leaflet of the mitral valve and Unilateral movement of the mitral valve anterior and posterior leaflets. Simulation By Echocardiography Online Simulator MyEchocardiography.com

Two Dimensional Echocardiography (B-Mode)

From the early stages of mitral stenosis, in the diastole phase, there is a dome-shaped bulging of the anterior leaflet of the mitral valve (towards the septum), which is caused by an increase in pressure on its unfixed part (Left parasternal view, the long axis of the heart).

In the later stages of mitral stenosis, the valve leaflets thicken and become rigid. Fusion of the leaflets and restriction of movement are often observed. From the left parasternal position, the short axis of the heart, there is a decrease in the area of the mitral orifice, which takes the form of an ellipsoid or gap. There is an increase in the size of the left atrium.

Increased pressure in the pulmonary circulation causes hypertrophy and dilatation of the right heart. The hepatic veins and inferior vena cava can be dilated.

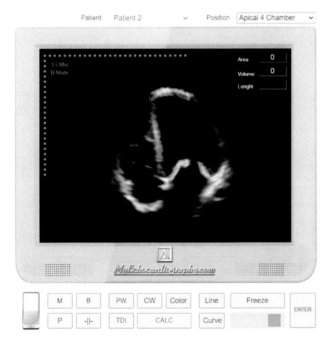

Apical 4 chamber view. 2D Echocardiography. Mitral Stenosis. Thick and rigid mitral valve leaflets. *Simulation By Echocardiography Online Simulator* MyEchocardiography.com

Spectral Doppler (PW, CW)

- Increased early transmitral diastolic flow velocity - caused by the increased pressure gradient between LA and LV.
- Spectrogram extension - caused by a reduction of the fall of the diastolic filling rate.

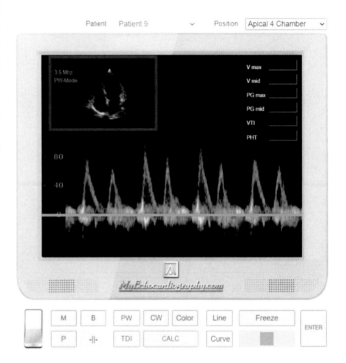

Apical 4 Chamber View. PW Doppler. Normal transmitral Diastolic Flow. Simulation By Echocardiography Online Simulator MyEchocardiography.com

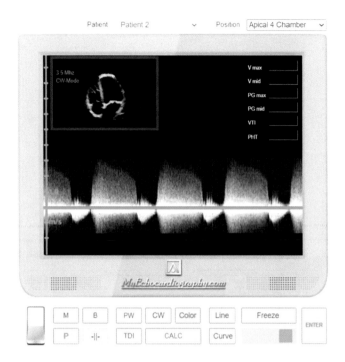

Patient   Patient 2   ⌄   Position   Apical 4 Chamber   ⌄

3 5 Mhz
CW-Mode

V max _____
V mid _____
PG max _____
PG mid _____
VTI _____
PHT _____

MyEchocardiography.com

| M | B | PW | CW | Color | Line | Freeze | |
| P | -\|\|- | TDI | CALC | | Curve | | ENTER |

Apical 4 Chamber View. CW Doppler. Mitral stenosis. Increase in velocity of early transmitral diastolic flow and spectrogram extension. Simulation By Echocardiography Online Simulator MyEchocardiography.com

Methods of measurement of the Mitral Valve Area (MVA)

- MVA Tracing
- PISA
- PHT
- Mitral Valve Area (MVA) by Continuity Equation
- Mean Pressure Gradient (PG mean)

MITRAL VALVE AREA BY TRACING

The area of the mitral orifice is measured planimetrically using two-dimensional echocardiography from the left parasternal position, the short axis of the heart at the level of the mitral valve (at the moment of maximum opening of the leaflets).

The contour of the orifice is outlined with the cursor (tracing). The ultrasound device will automatically calculate the area.

Assessment of mitral stenosis using planimetry can be divided into the following steps:

• The image must first be acquired from the Left Parasternal Position at the Level of the Papillary Muscles.
• Then rotate the transducer until the end of the mitral leaflets is imaged. In this case, the area of the mitral orifice is minimal.
• Freeze the image in the early diastole phase.
• Make a tracing of the mitral valve along the internal borders.

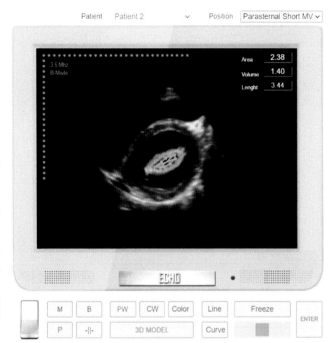

Left Parasternal View, Short axis at the level of the mitral valve. Tracing of the Mitral Valve. Simulation By Echocardiography Online Simulator MyEchocardiography.com

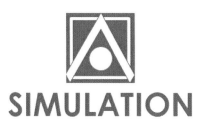

SIMULATION
MITRAL VALVE AREA MEASUREMENT BY TRACING

Echocardiography Online Simulator
MyEchocardiography.com

- Go to the link https://simulation.myechocardiography.com/

- Run Echocardiography Online Simulator using the **On/Off** Button

- Choose the patient 2 from the list **<<Patient>>**

- Choose **<<Parasternal Short MV>>** (Left Parasternal View, Short axis At the Level of Mitral Valve) from the List **<<Positions>>** or find the position with **3D Transducer**

- Click the button **<<Freeze>>** to freeze image. Using Slider find the frame of maximum opening of the mitral valve.

- Click Button **<<Calculations>>** Click Tab **<<MV St >>** Click the Radio Button **<<MVA>>**

- Click the button **<<Curve>>** trace around inner side of the Mitral Valve.

- Click the button **<<Enter>>**

- Click the button << R >> to see the results.

- To change the patient, click the **On/Off** Button

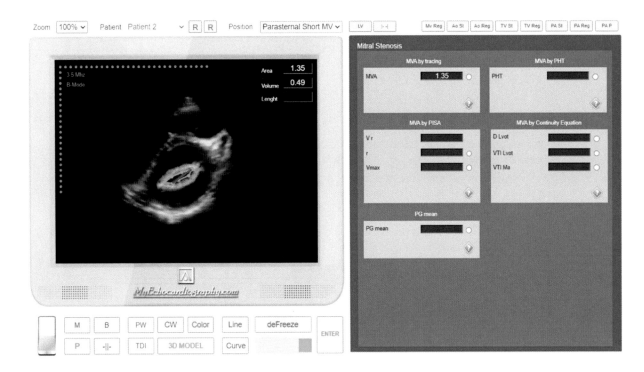

Left Parasternal View, Short axis at the level of the mitral valve. Tracing of the Mitral Valve. Simulation By Echocardiography Online Simulator MyEchocardiography.com

https://youtu.be/DrmJgCxX92U

MITRAL STENOSIS

MITRAL VALVE AREA BY PHT (Pressure Half-time)

The time at which the maximum gradient of the transmitral diastolic flow is halved can be used to measure Mitral Valve Area (MVA). It is the so-called pressure half-time (T ½) or PHT (Pressure Half-time).

Empirically, if the Mitral Valve Area (MVA) is 1 cm2, then the Pressure Half-Time (PHT) is 220 s. From here, we can find the MVA:

$$MVA = \frac{220}{PHT}$$

MVA - Mitral Valve Area. PHT - Pressure Half-Time

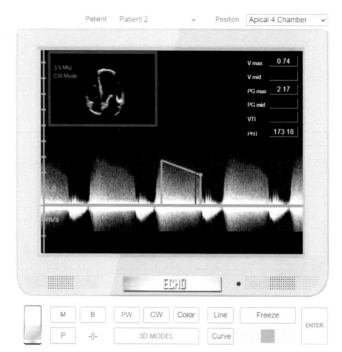

Apical 4 Chamber View. CW doppler. Transmitral diastolic flow. Measurement of the Pressure Half-Time (PHT). Simulation By Echocardiography Online Simulator MyEchocardiography.com

Assessment of mitral stenosis by the Mitral Valve Area (MVA):

- Mild > 1.5 cm2
- Moderate 1.0 - 1.5 cm2
- Severe < 1.0 cm2

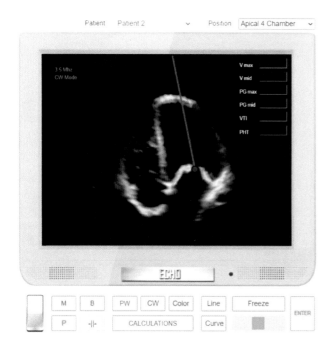

Apical 4 Chamber View. Sample Volume position for examining the transmitral diastolic flow. Simulation By Echocardiography Online Simulator MyEchocardiography.com

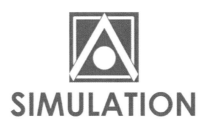

SIMULATION

MITRAL VALVE AREA MEASUREMENT BY PHT

Echocardiography Online Simulator
MyEchocardiography.com

- Go to the link https://simulation.myechocardiography.com/

- Run Echocardiography Online Simulator using the **On/Off** Button

- Choose the patient 2 from the list **<<Patient>>**

- Choose **<<Apical 4 Chamber>>** (Apical For Chamber View) from the List **<<Positions>>** or find the position with **3D Transducer**

- Click the button **<<CW>>** Place the "Sample Volume" in the Mitral Valve and click.

- Click Button **<<Calculations>>** Click Tab **<<MV St >>** Click the Radio Button **<<PHT>>** and perform Spectral Doppler Measurements (see Lesson 8)

- Click the button **<<Enter>>**

- Click the button << R >> to see the results.

- To change the patient, click the **On/Off** Button

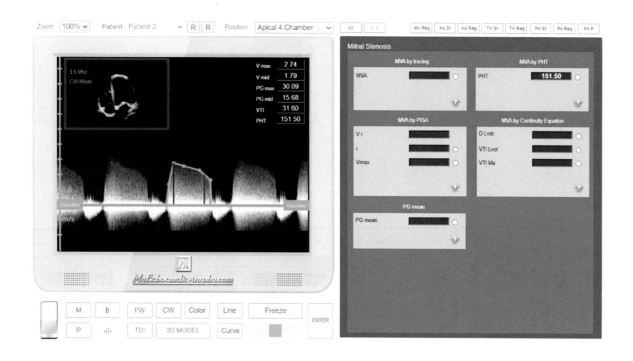

Apical 4 Chamber View. CW doppler. Transmitral diastolic flow. Measurement of the Pressure Half-Time (PHT). Simulation By Echocardiography Online Simulator _MyEchocardiography.com_

https://youtu.be/5a0CgWuF05s

MITRAL STENOSIS

MITRAL VALVE AREA (CONTINUITY EQUATION)

The Continuity Equation can be used to calculate the area of the mitral valve and estimate the degree of stenosis:

$$MVA = \frac{CSA_{LVOT} \times VTI_{Ao}}{VTI_{MV}}$$

CSA_{LVOT} - Cross-Sectional Area of LVOT. VTI_{Ao} - **VTI** of the transaortic flow. VTI_{MV} - **VTI** of the transmitral flow.

To calculate the cross-sectional area of LVOT (**CSA_{LVOT}**), it is necessary to measure the D - diameter of the Left Ventricular Outflow Tract (LVOT).

$$CSA_{LVOT} = D^2_{LVOT} \times 0.785$$

D - LVOT diameter.

Assessment of mitral stenosis by the Mitral Valve Area (MVA):

- Mild > 1.5 cm2
- Moderate 1.0 - 1.5 cm2
- Severe < 1.0 cm2

$$MVA = \frac{220}{PHT}$$

MVA - Mitral Valve Area. PHT - Pressure Half-Time

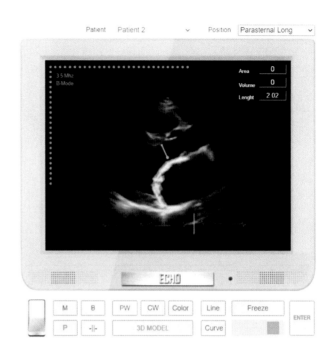

Left Parasternal View, the Long axis of LV. Measurement of the LVOT diameter. Simulation By Echocardiography Online Simulator MyEchocardiography.com

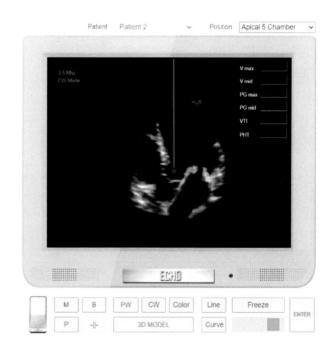

Apical 5 chamber view. CW Doppler. Control Volume in LVOT. Simulation By Echocardiography Online Simulator MyEchocardiography.com

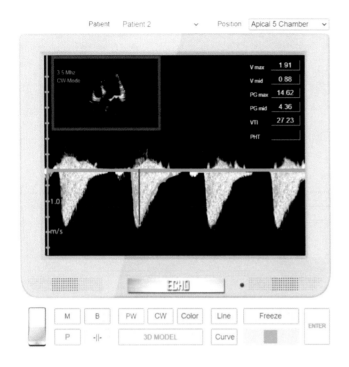

Apical 5 chamber view. CW doppler. Measurement of the VTI LVOT. Simulation By Echocardiography Online Simulator MyEchocardiography.com

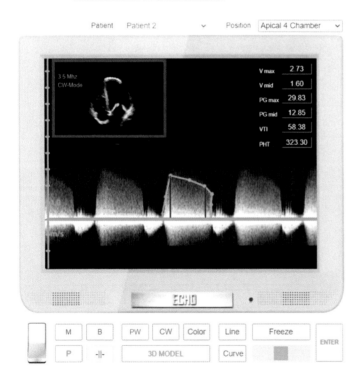

Apical 4 chamber view. CW doppler. VTI MV measurement. Simulation By Echocardiography Online Simulator MyEchocardiography.com

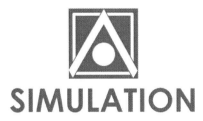

SIMULATION
MITRAL VALVE AREA MEASUREMENT BY CONTINUITY EQUATION

Echocardiography Online Simulator
MyEchocardiography.com

- Go to the link https://simulation.myechocardiography.com/

- Run Echocardiography Online Simulator using the **On/Off** Button

- Choose the patient 2 from the list **<<Patient>>**

- Choose **<< Parasternal Long >>** (Left Parasternal View, Long axis of LV) from the List **<<Positions>>** or find the position with **3D Transducer**

- Click the button **<<Freeze>>** to freeze image.

- Click Button **<<Calculations>>** Click Tab **<<MV st >>** Click Radio Button **<<D Lvot>>** (Calculator MVA by Continuity equation).

- Click the button **<<Line>>** Measure linear size of **Left Ventricular Outflow Tract (LVOT).**

- Click the button **<<Enter>>**

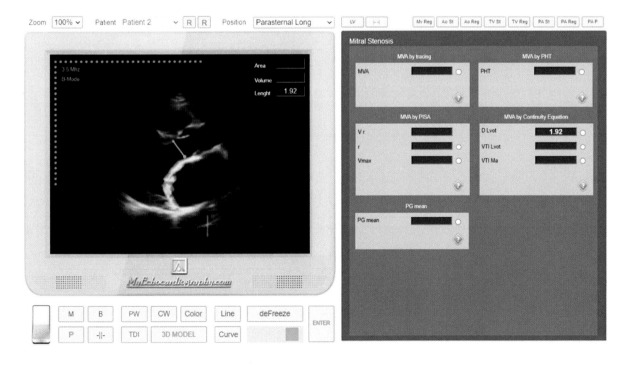

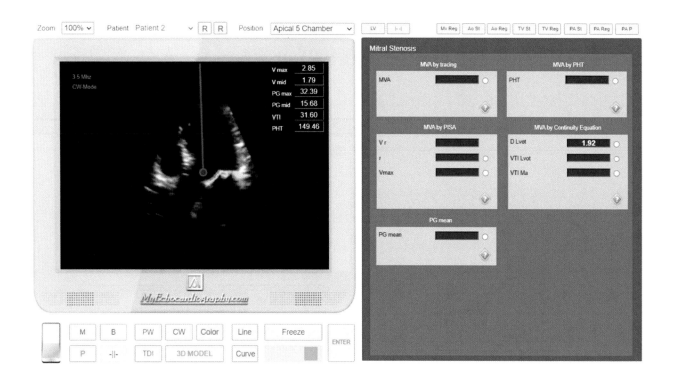

Apical 5 chamber view. CW Doppler. "Sample Volume" in LVOT. Simulation By Echocardiography Online Simulator MyEchocardiography.com

- From the List **<<Positions>>** Choose **Apical 5 Chamber** or <u>find the same position with</u> **3D Transducer.** in the Tab **<<MV st >>** Click Radio Button **<<VTI Lvot>>**
- Click the button **<<CW>>** to start CW doppler examination. Place the "Sample Volume" in the LVOT (Left Ventricular Outflow Tractact) and **Click**.
- Click the button **<<Curve>>** place points around spectrogram of the LVOT flow. (see Lesson 8)
- Click the button **<<Enter>>**

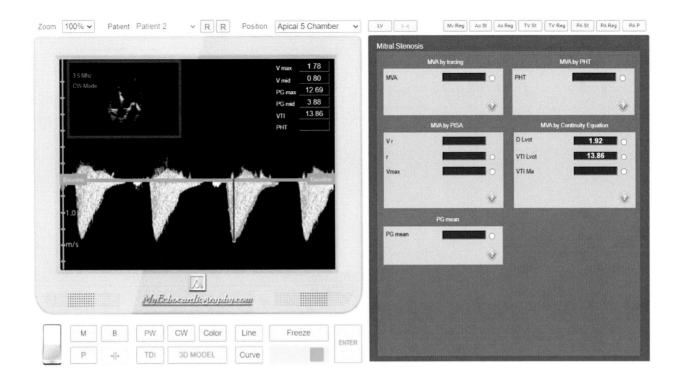

Apical 5 chamber view. CW doppler. Measurement of the VTI LVOT. Simulation By Echocardiography Online Simulator MyEchocardiography.com

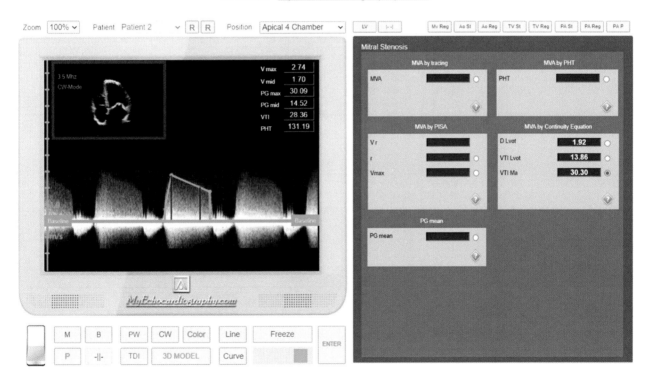

Apical 4 chamber view. CW doppler. VTImv measurement. Simulation By Echocardiography Online Simulator MyEchocardiography.com

- Choose **<<Apical 4 Chamber>>** (Apical For Chamber View) from the List **<<Positions>>** or <u>find the position with</u> **3D Transducer**
- Click the button **<<CW>>** Place the "Sample Volume" in the Mitral Valve and click.
- Click the Radio Button **<<VTI mv>>** and perform Spectral Doppler Measurements (see Lesson 8)
- Click the button **<<Enter>>**
- Click the button << R >> to see the results.
- To change the patient, click the **On/Off** Button

https://youtu.be/9zu-w833u8w

DEGREE OF MITRAL STENOSIS BY MEAN PRESSURE GRADIENT

For mitral stenosis assessment, measuring the pressure difference between the left atrium and the ventricle (in the apical four-chamber position) is necessary.

Both maximum and mean pressure gradients can be measured.

PGmax - Maximum flow gradient, measured at the maximum point of velocity.

PGmid - (Mean Gradient) - The sum of the gradients measured every 2 seconds, divided by the number of measurements.

For PGmax calculation, we need the maximum flow rate at point E. Using the Bernoulli formula ultrasound device will calculate the maximum pressure gradient:

$$\triangle p = 4V^2$$

V - maximum flow rate.

For the mean pressure gradient (PGmid), we need to trace the spectrogram of the transmitral diastolic flow. The ultrasound device will calculate the mean pressure gradient.

The mean gradient is the relevant hemodynamic finding. The maximal gradient is of little interest as it derives from peak mitral velocity, which is influenced by left atrial compliance and LV diastolic function.

Assessment of mitral stenosis by the mean pressure gradient (PGmid)

- Mild < 5 mmHg
- Moderate 5 - 10 mmHg
- Severe > 10 mmHg

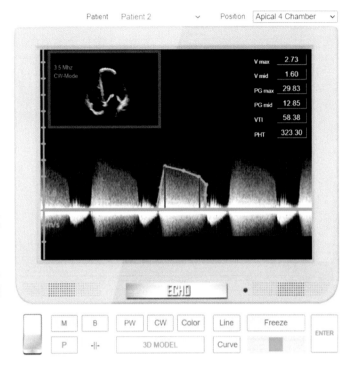

Apical 4 Chamber View. CW doppler. Transmitral diastolic flow. Measurement of the Pressure Mean Gradient. Simulation By Echocardiography Online Simulator *MyEchocardiography.com*

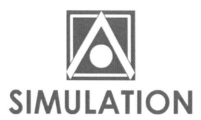

SIMULATION
DEGREE OF MITRAL STENOSIS BY MEAN PRESSURE GRADIENT

Echocardiography Online Simulator
MyEchocardiography.com

- Go to the link https://simulation.myechocardiography.com/

- Run Echocardiography Online Simulator using the **On/Off** Button

- Choose the patient 2 from the list **<<Patient>>**

- Choose **<<Apical 4 Chamber>>** (Apical For Chamber View) from the List **<<Positions>>** or find the position with **3D Transducer**

- Click the button **<<CW>>** Place the "Sample Volume" in the Mitral Valve and click.

- Click Button **<<Calculations>>** Click Tab **<<MV St >>** Click the Radio Button **<<PG mean>>** and perform Spectral Doppler Measurements (see Lesson 8)

- Click the button **<<Enter>>**

- Click the button << **R** >> to see the results.

- To change the patient, click the **On/Off** Button

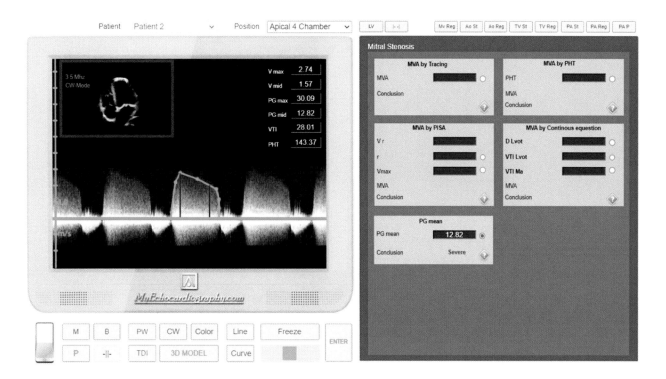

Apical 4 Chamber View. CW doppler. Transmitral diastolic flow. Measurement of the Pressure Mean Gradient. Simulation By Echocardiography Online Simulator MyEchocardiography.com

https://youtu.be/wRpuD2WNmsw

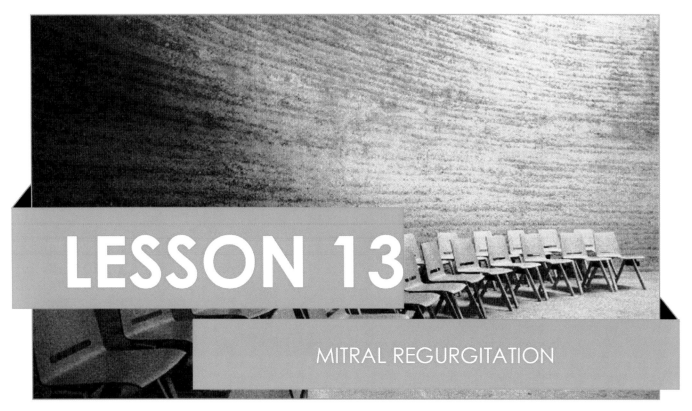

LESSON 13

MITRAL REGURGITATION

One and two-dimensional Echocardiography

There are no direct echocardiographic signs of mitral regurgitation using 1D and 2D Echocardiography.

The only relatively reliable finding can be the Incomplete closure of the valve on a one-dimensional echocardiogram, which is rarely seen.

Non-specific symptoms: Increase in the size of the left atrium. LV Myocardial hypertrophy and dilatation.

Color Doppler

The most informative method is Color Doppler. Regurgitation flow is observed in the systolic phase, which returns to the left atrium (away from the transducer) and is encoded in blue. Its size and volume depend on the severity of regurgitation.

Slight regurgitation can be identified in 40-60% of healthy people (physiological regurgitation).

The best positions for evaluation: Apical 4 Chamber, Apical 2 Chamber Views, and the Left Parasternal View, long axis.

MITRAL REGURGITATION

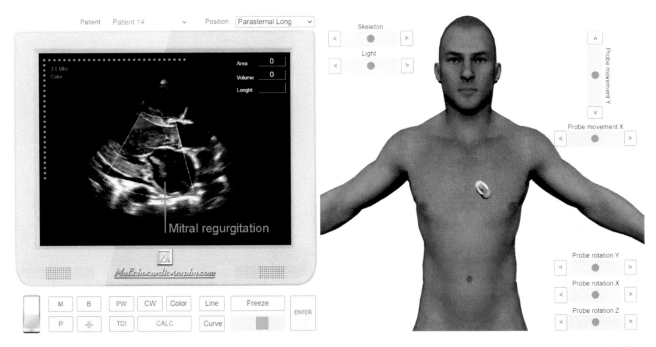

Left Parasternal View, the long axis. Color Doppler. Mitral regurgitation. One dimensional Echocardiography (m-mode). Normal Mitral Valve. Simulation By Echocardiography Online Simulator MyEchocardiography.com

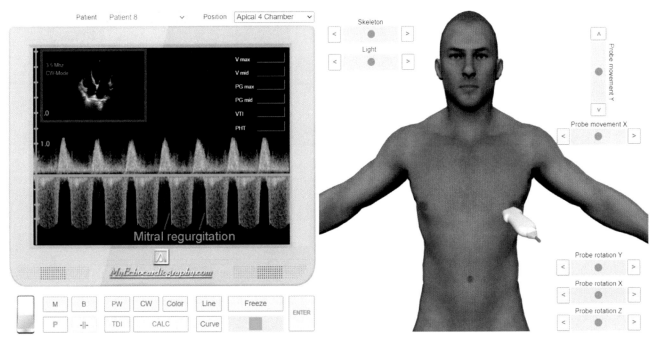

Apical 4 Chamber View. CW Doppler. Mitral regurgitation. *Simulation By Echocardiography Online Simulator MyEchocardiography.com*

MITRAL REGURGITATION

Spectral Doppler (PW, CW)

The best positions for evaluation: Apical 4 Chamber and Apical 2 Chamber Views. To find the regurgitation and determine the depth of its penetration, the sample volume has to be moved at different distances from the mitral valve.

The regurgitation flow is visible on the spectrogram as a characteristic spectrum directed downward from the baseline. The flow captures the entire systole (from the mitral valve's closing to the aortic valve's opening).

Methods of assessment severity of the mitral Regurgitation:

- Regurgiration Area
- Reg Area / LA area
- PISA
- Regurgitation volume and fraction (CV method)
- Vena Contracta

DEGREE OF MITRAL REGURGITATION BY JET AREA OR JET AREA/LA AREA RATIO

Using the color Doppler, it is possible to assess the degree of mitral regurgitation by the regurgitation area and its percentage ratio with the area of the left atrium.

JET AREA

Jet has to be measured in Color Doppler mode using apical positions (Tracing around the regurgitation jet). Grading the severity of chronic mitral regurgitation by jet area:
- Mild - Small, central, narrow, often brief (usually < 4 cm2).
- Moderate - Variable.
- Severe - Large central jet (usually > 10 cm2) or eccentric wall-impinging jet of variable size

JET AREA/LA AREA RATIO

Jet has to be measured in Color Doppler mode using apical positions (Tracing around the regurgitation jet). The Left Atrium area has to be measured in the same echocardiography view.

Grading the severity of chronic mitral regurgitation by jet area/LA area ratio:

- Mild - Small, central, narrow, often brief (usually < 20% of LA area).
- Moderate - Variable.
- Severe - Large central jet (>50% of LA) or eccentric wall-impinging jet of variable size.

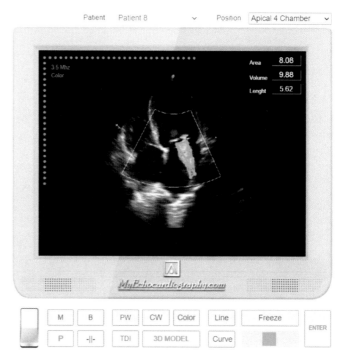

Apical 4 chamber View. Mitral regurgitation. Regurgitation jet area measurement. Simulation By Echocardiography Online Simulator MyEchocardiography.com

---

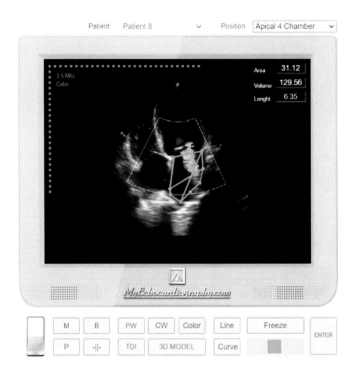

| Patient | Patient 8 | ∨ | Position | Apical 4 Chamber ∨ |

Area	31.12
Volume	129.56
Lenght	6 35

3 5 Mhz
Color

MyEchocardiography.com

| M | B | PW | CW | Color | Line | Freeze | ENTER |
| P | -\|\|- | TDI | 3D MODEL | Curve | | | |

Apical 4 chamber View. Mitral regurgitation. LA area measurement. Simulation By Echocardiography Online Simulator MyEchocardiography.com

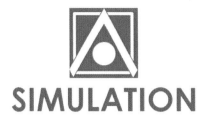

SIMULATION

DEGREE OF MITRAL REGURGITATION BY JET AREA OR JET AREA/LA AREA RATIO

Echocardiography Online Simulator
MyEchocardiography.com

- Go to the link https://simulation.myechocardiography.com/
- Run Echocardiography Online Simulator using the **On/Off** Button
- Choose the patient 8 from the list **<<Patient>>**
- Choose **<<Apical 4 chamber>>** from the List **<<Positions>>** or find the position with **3D Transducer**
- Using **Slider** find the frame of maximum regurgitation size.

JET AREA

- find the calculator **<<Regurgitation Area>>** Click Radio Button **<<Area>>**
- Click the button **<<Curve>>** place points around regurgitation jet.
- Click the button **<<Enter>>**
- Click the button << R >> to see the results.
- To change the patient, click the **On/Off** Button

JET AREA / LA AREA

- After the above step, find the calculator **<< Area reg / Area LA>>** Click Radio Button **<< Area LA>>**
- Click the button **<<Curve>>** place points around inner side of the Left Atrium.
- Click the button **<<Enter>>**
- Click the button << R >> to see the results.
- To change the patient, click the **On/Off** Button

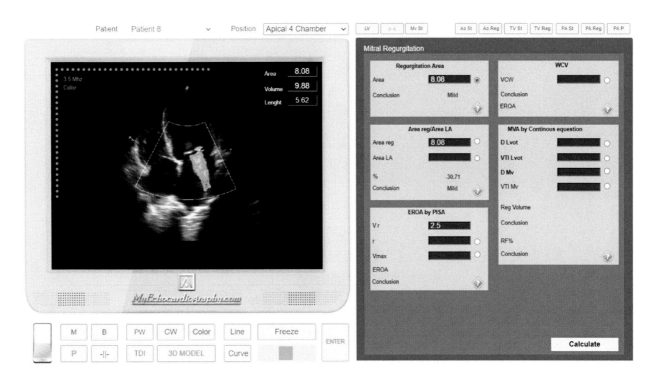

Apical 4 chamber View. Mitral regurgitation. Regurgitation jet area measurement. Simulation By Echocardiography Online Simulator MyEchocardiography.com

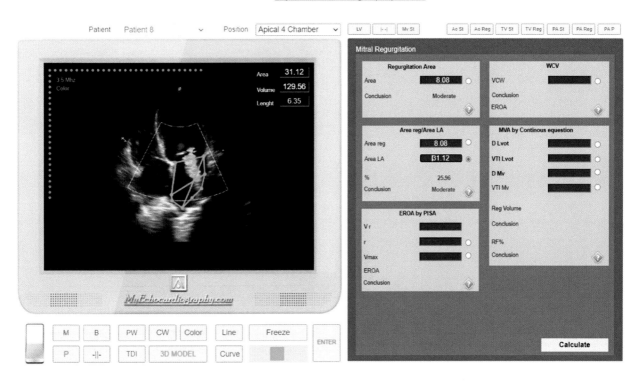

Apical 4 chamber View. Mitral regurgitation. LA area measurement. Simulation By Echocardiography Online Simulator MyEchocardiography.com

https://www.youtube.com/watch?v=F6gOVUW58Ls

DEGREE OF MITRAL REGURGITATION BY FLOW CONVERGENCE METHOD (PISA)

The radius of the proximal zone (PISA - Proximal Isovelosity surface Area) is a parameter characterizing the severity of regurgitation, determined by color Doppler. PISA is part of the color spectrum on the ventricular side of the mitral valve.

The formation of the flow of regurgitation begins before entering the left atrium. The more regurgitation, the more area PISA occupies in the left ventricle. To measure the radius of the proximal zone, the regurgitation flow velocity must exceed the Nyquist limit and turn red. We need to increase the image size and decrease the Nyquist limit to do this.

PISA is made up of several layers. Each of them corresponds to a specific flow rate. The volumetric regurgitation rate can be calculated based on the assumption that all of the regurgitation flow will be on the other side of the valve and based on the principle of mass invariance.

$$Q = 2\pi r^2 V_r$$

r - the radius of the proximal zone of the flow of regurgitation. Vr - Minimum speed when the Doppler spectrum is distorted (exceeds the Nyquist limit).

The area of the regurgitation orifice is calculated by the following formula:

$$EROA = \frac{Q}{V_{max}} = \frac{2\pi r^2 V_r}{V_{max}}$$

Vmax - Maximum regurgitation flow rate. V r- Nyquist limit.

Measurement can be divided into the next stages:

- Align insonation beam with the flow, usually in apical views; zoomed view
- Lower the color Doppler baseline in the direction of the jet.
- Look for the hemispheric shape to guide the best low Nyquist limit
- Look for the need for angle correction if the flow convergence zone is nonplanar
- Measure PISA radius at roughly the same time as the CW jet peak velocity

Degree of Mitral Regurgitation by EROA (cm2)

- Mild < 0.20
- Mild-Moderate 0.20 - 0.29
- Moderate-severe 0.30 - 0.39
- Severe > 0.40

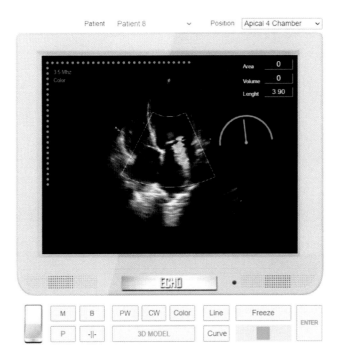

Apical 4 Chamber view. Color Doppler. Degree of Mitral Regurgitation by Proximal Isovelocity Surface Area (PISA). Simulation By Echocardiography Online Simulator MyEchocardiography.com

MITRAL REGURGITATION

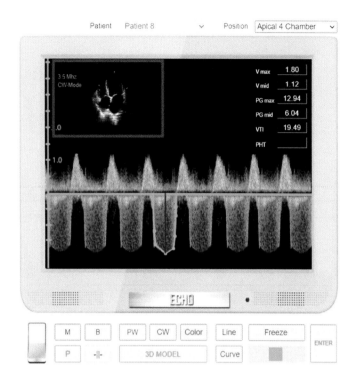

| Patient | Patient 8 | ⌄ | Position | Apical 4 Chamber | ⌄ |

V max	1.80
V mid	1.12
PG max	12.94
PG mid	6.04
VTI	19.49
PHT	

3.5 Mhz
CW-Mode

.0

1.0

ECHO

| M | B | PW | CW | Color | Line | Freeze | ENTER |
| P | -||- | 3D MODEL | Curve | | |

Apical 4 Chamber view, CW Doppler. Mitral Regurgitation Vmax (maximum velocity) Assessment. Simulation By Echocardiography Online Simulator MyEchocardiography.com

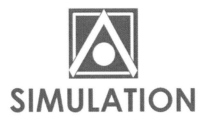

SIMULATION

DEGREE OF MITRAL REGURGITATION BY FLOW CONVERGENCE METHOD (PISA)

Echocardiography Online Simulator
MyEchocardiography.com

- Go to the link https://simulation.myechocardiography.com/
- Run Echocardiography Online Simulator using the **On/Off** Button
- Choose the patient 8 from the list **<<Patient>>**
- Choose **<<Apical 4 chamber>>** from the List **<<Positions>>** or find the position with **3D Transducer**
- Click the button **<<Color>>**
- Click the button **<<Freeze>>** to freeze image. Click the Button **<< - | | - >>** and increase zoom level. Using Slider find the best frame for PISA measurement. The Nyquist Limit is set to 2.5.
- Click Button **<<Calculations>>** Click Tab **<<MV Reg>>** Click Radio Button **<<r>>** (Calculator **EROA by PISA**).
- Click the button **<<Line>>** measure radius of the PISA.
- Click the button **<<Enter>>**
- Click the button << R >> to see the results.
- To change the patient, click the **On/Off** Button

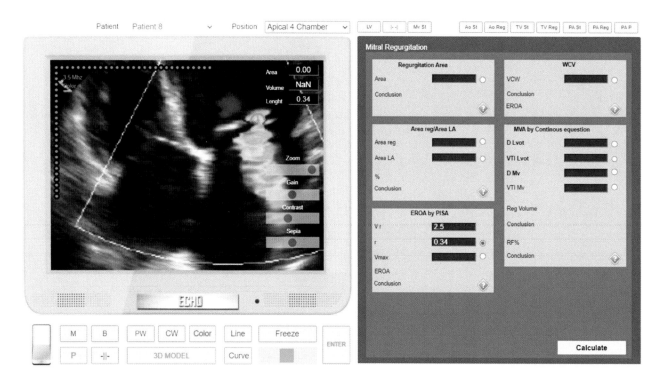

Apical 4 Chamber view. Color Doppler. Degree of Mitral Regurgitation by Proximal Isovelocity Surface Area (PISA). Zoomed image. Simulation By Echocardiography Online Simulator MyEchocardiography.com

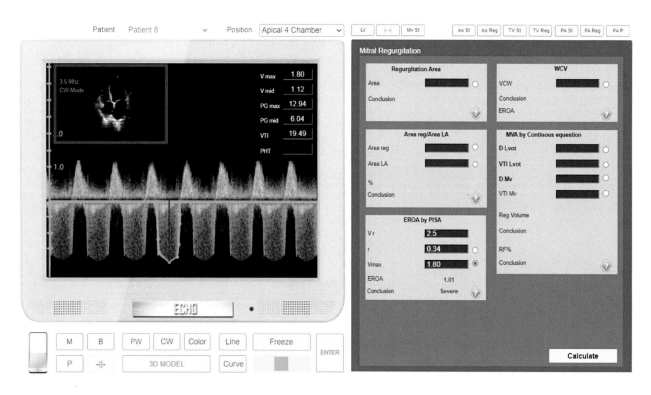

Apical 4 Chamber view, CW Doppler. Mitral Regurgitation Vmax (maximum velocity) Assessment. Simulation By Echocardiography Online Simulator MyEchocardiography.com

https://youtu.be/y2PVNq6dHXY

DEGREE OF MITRAL REGURGITATION BY REGURGITATION VOLUME AND FRACTION

The volume of mitral regurgitation is the difference between the transmitral flow and the flow in the outflow tract of the left ventricle.

$$RV = SV_{mv} - SV_{LVOT}$$

RV - regurgitation volume. SVmv - transmitral stroke Volume. SVLVOT - LVOT Stroke Volume.

To calculate the transmitral Stroke Volume (SV), measuring the mitral annulus's D-diameter and VTI of the transmitral flow is necessary.

$$SV_{MV} = D_{MV}^2 \times 0.785 \times VTI_{MV}$$

D - diameter of the mitral annulus. VTIMV - VTI of the transmitral flow.

To calculate the stroke volume through the outflow tract of the left ventricle, it is necessary to measure the D-diameter of the LVOT and the VTI of the flow in the outflow tract of the left ventricle (LVOT).

$$SV_{LVOT} = D_{LVOT}^2 \times 0.785 \times VTI_{LVOT}$$

D - diameter of the LVOT. VTILVOT - VTI of the LVOT flow

- LVOT diameter measured at the annulus in systole and pulsed Doppler from apical views at the same site
- Mitral annulus measured at mid diastole; pulsed Doppler at the annulus level in diastole
- Total LV SV can be measured by the pulsed Doppler technique at the mitral annulus or by the difference between LV end-diastolic and end-systolic volumes.
- LV volumes are best measured in 3D. Contrast may be needed to trace endocardial borders better. If 3D is not feasible, use the 2D method of disks.

Assessment of mitral regurgitation by the regurgitation volume:

- Mild < 30
- Mild-Moderate 30 - 44
- Moderate-severe 45 - 59
- Severe > 60

The following formula determines the regurgitation fraction (RF%):

$$RF(\%) = \frac{RV}{SV_{mv}}$$

Assessment of mitral regurgitation by the regurgitation fraction (RF%):

- Mild < 30
- Mild-Moderate 30 - 39
- Moderate-severe 40 - 49
- Severe > 50

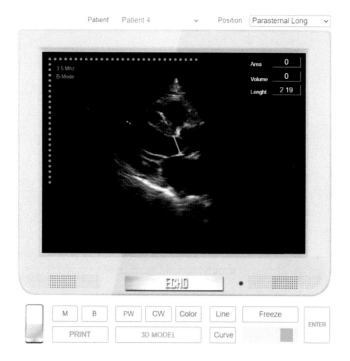

Left Parasternal View. The long axis of LV. Measurement of the Left Ventricular Outflow Tract (LVOT) diameter. Simulation By Echocardiography Online Simulator MyEchocardiography.com

MITRAL REGURGITATION

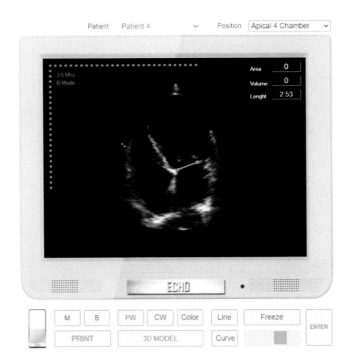

Apical 4 chamber view. Measurement of the Mitral Annulus Diameter. *Simulation By Echocardiography Online Simulator* *MyEchocardiography.com*

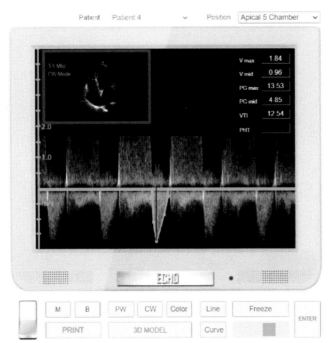

Apical 5 chamber view. CW Doppler. VTI LVOT measurement. *Simulation By Echocardiography Online Simulator* *MyEchocardiography.com*

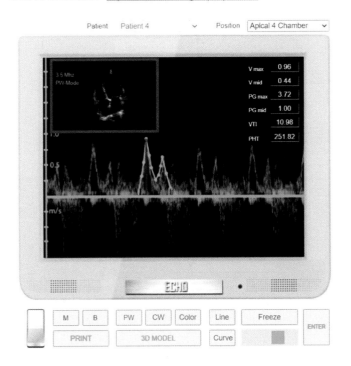

Apical 4 chamber view. PW Doppler. VTI mv measurement. *Simulation By Echocardiography Online Simulator* *MyEchocardiography.com*

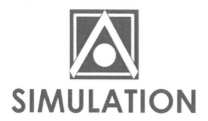

SIMULATION

DEGREE OF MITRAL REGURGITATION BY REGURGITATION VOLUME AND FRACTION

Echocardiography Online Simulator
MyEchocardiography.com

- Go to the link https://simulation.myechocardiography.com/

- Run Echocardiography Online Simulator using the **On/Off** Button

- From the List **<<Patients>>** Choose **Patient 4** (User can Choose other patients with mitral regurgitation as well).

- From the List **<<Positions>>** Choose **Parasternal Long** (Left Parasternal View, Long axis of LV). or find the same position with **3D Transducer**.

- Click the button **<<Freeze>>** to freeze image.

- Click Button **<<Calculations>>** Click Tab **<<MV Reg>>** Click Radio Button **<<D Lvot>>**

- Click the button **<<Line>>** Measure linear size of **Left Ventricular Outflow Tract (LVOT).** See Linear measurements.

- Click the button **<<Enter>>**

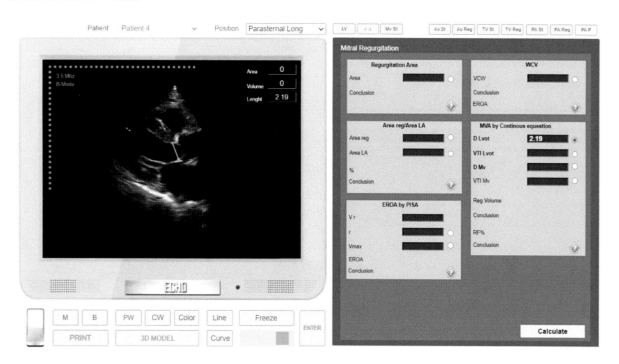

Left Parasternal View. The long axis of LV. Measurement of the Left Ventricular Outflow Tract (LVOT) diameter.
Simulation By Echocardiography Online Simulator MyEchocardiography.com

- From the List **<<Positions>>** Choose **Apical 4 Chamber** or <u>find the same position with</u> **3D Transducer**.
- Click the button **<<Freeze>>** to freeze image.
- Click Button **<<Calculations>>** Click Tab **<<MV Reg>>** Click Radio Button **<<D mv>>**
- Click the button **<<Line>>** Measure **Mitral Anullus Diameter**. <u>See Linear measurements.</u>
- Click the button **<<Enter>>**

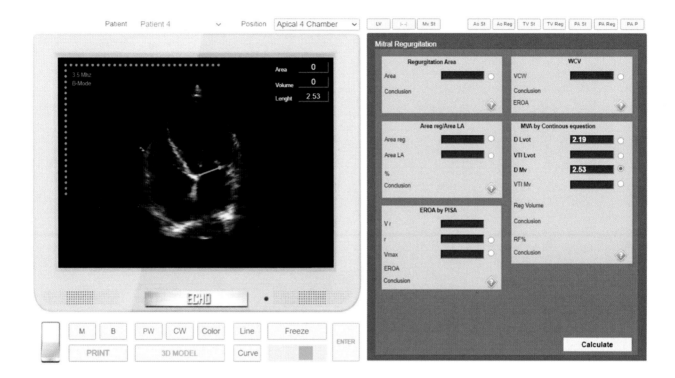

Apical 4 chamber view. Measurement of the Mitral Annulus Diameter. Simulation By Echocardiography Online Simulator *MyEchocardiography.com*

- In the Tab **<<MV Reg>>** Click Radio Button **<<VTI mv>>**
- Click the button **<<PW>>** to start Pulse Wave Doppler examination. Place Control Volume Between Mitral Valve Leaflets and **Click**.
- Click the button **<<Curve>>** place points around spectrogram of trans-mitral diastolic flow.
- Click the button **<<Enter>>**

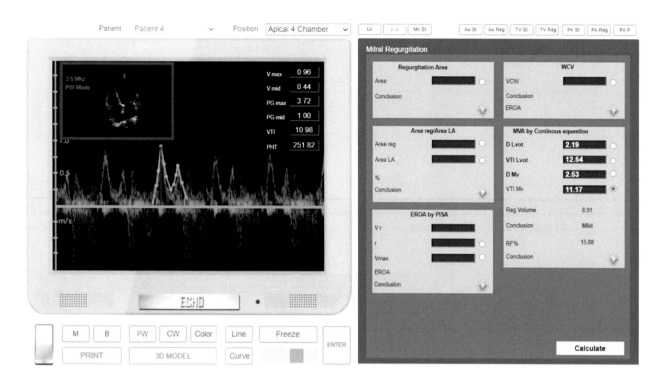

Apical 4 chamber view. PW Doppler. VTI mv measurement. Simulation By Echocardiography Online Simulator MyEchocardiography.com

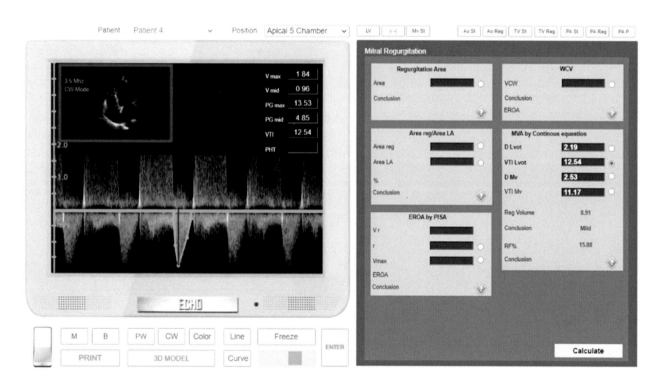

Apical 5 chamber view. CW Doppler. VTI LVOT measurement. Simulation By Echocardiography Online Simulator MyEchocardiography.com

https://youtu.be/4qF88qt3K7M

DEGREE OF MITRAL REGURGITATION BY VENA CONTRACTA WIDTH (VCW)

Vena Contracta - this is the width of the flow at the site of its formation, the so-called neck of the regurgitation, the narrowest point of the flow, at the ends of the leaflets of the closed mitral valve.

Vena Contracta Width (VCW) can be used to assess the severity of regurgitation:

Vena Contracta Width (VCW) can be used to assess the severity of regurgitation:

- Mild - Vena Contracta < 0.3 cm.
- Moderate - Intermediate.
- Severe - Vena Contracta > 0.7 cm (>0.8 for biplane. For average between apical two and four-chamber views).

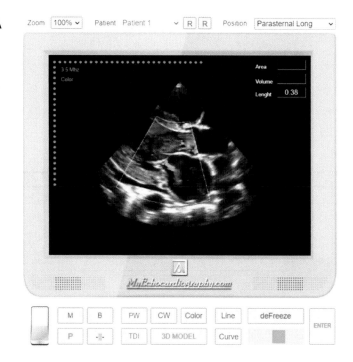

Left Parasternal View, the Long axis of LV, Mitral regurgitation. VCW measurement. Simulation By Echocardiography Online Simulator MyEchocardiography.com

Vena Contracta can also be used to determine the effective area of the regurgitation orifice (EROA):

$$EROA = \pi \left(\frac{VCW}{2} \right)^2$$

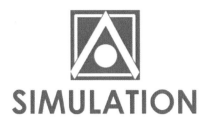

SIMULATION
DEGREE OF MITRAL REGURGITATION BY VENA CONTRACTA WIDTH (VCW)
Echocardiography Online Simulator
MyEchocardiography.com

- Go to the link https://simulation.myechocardiography.com/
- Run Echocardiography Online Simulator using the **On/Off** Button
- Choose the patient 4 from the list **<<Patient>>**
- Choose **<<Apical 4 chamber>>** from the List **<<Positions>>** or find the position with **3D Transducer**
- Click the button **<<Color>>** to run **Color Doppler**.
- Click the button **<<Freeze>>** to freeze image. Using **Slider** find the frame of maximum regurgitation size.
- Click Button **<<Calculations>>** Click Tab **<<MV Reg >>** Click Radio Button **<<VCW>>**
- Click the button **<<Line>>** Measure linear size of VCW.
- Click the button **<<Enter>>**
- Click the button **<< R >>** to see the results.
- To change the patient, click the **On/Off** Button

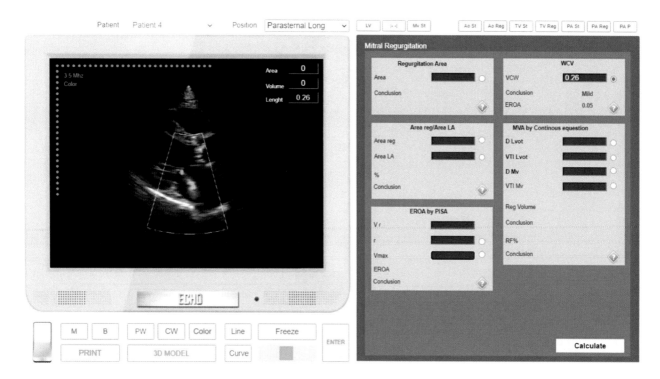

Left Parasternal View, the Long axis of LV, Mitral regurgitation. VCW measurement. Simulation By Echocardiography Online Simulator MyEchocardiography.com

https://youtu.be/JJvpEp66Osl

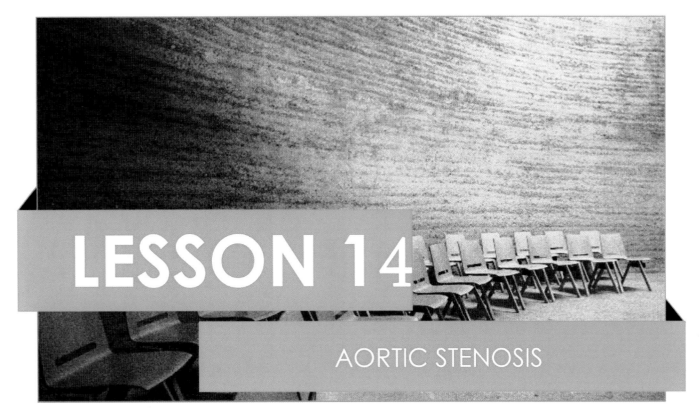

LESSON 14

AORTIC STENOSIS

One-dimensional Echocardiography

The examination must be done in the left parasternal position, on the long axis of the heart.

One-dimensional echocardiography will reveal changes in the structure and motion of the valve leaflets. There is a decrease in the amplitude of the systolic opening of the leaflets and their movement in one direction. It is worth noting that the hardening and thickening of the aortic valve also give us a similar picture even in the absence of hemodynamically significant stenosis, so a one-dimensional echocardiogram cannot be focused only on.

Two dimensional Echocardiography

A two-dimensional echocardiographic study should be performed on the short and long axis.

The number of leaflets, the amplitude of their movement (opening), thickness, and the presence of calcification should be evaluated.

A two-dimensional echocardiogram will reveal a decrease in the opening amplitude of the leaflets.
In the case of hemodynamically significant stenosis, such indirect signs as the post-stenotic expansion of the aorta, increase in the thickness and mass of the left ventricular wall, and increase in the size of the left atrium can be presented.

Mitral Regurgitation

- Aortic stenosis diagnosis.
- Degree of the Aortic Stenosis by Pic Velosity of the Stenotic Flow
- Degree of the Aortic Stenosis by Mean Pressure Gradient
- Degree of the Aortic Stenosis by Aortic Valve Area (AVA)

AORTIC STENOSIS

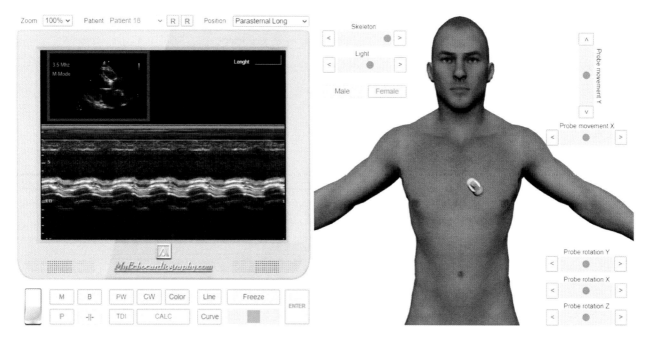

Left Parasternal View. The long axis. M-Mode. Aortic Stenosis. Simulation By Echocardiography Online Simulator MyEchocardiography.com

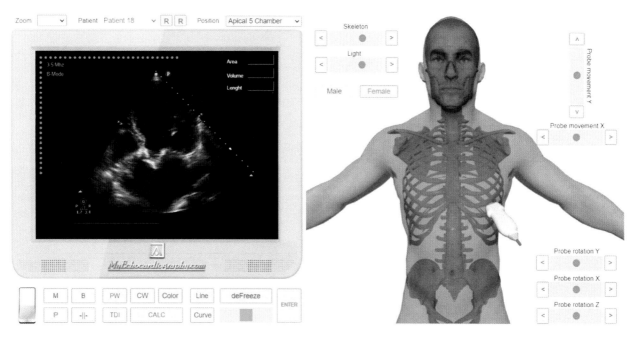

Apical 5 Chamber View. B-Mode. Aortic Stenosis. Simulation By Echocardiography Online Simulator MyEchocardiography.com

AORTIC STENOSIS

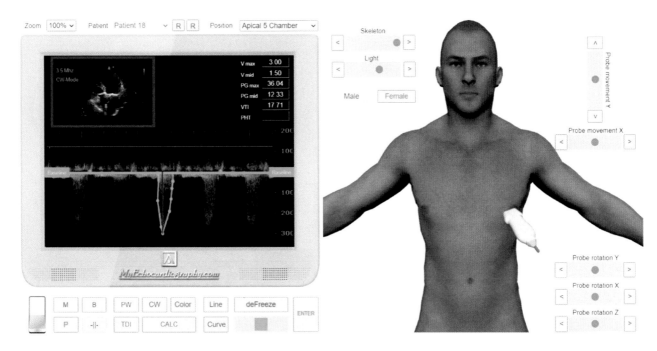

Apical 5 Chamber View. CW Doppler. Measurement of the Pic Velosity of the systolic flow and Mean pressure gradient. Aortic Stenosis. Simulation By Echocardiography Online Simulator MyEchocardiography.com

Spectral Doppler (PW, CW)

Continuous-wave and pulsed-wave spectral Doppler will reveal increased flow velocity beyond the aortic valve. Increased transaortic flow velocity is one of the most sensitive tests for aortic stenosis.

In spectral Doppler examination, the maximum flow velocity through the stenotic aortic valve is usually obtained from the apical five-chamber position. The ultrasound beam should be directed parallel to the stenotic flow.

The pressure gradient (pressure difference) between the left ventricle and the aorta is calculated using continuous wave Doppler.

Methods of assessment severity of the Aortic Stenosis:

- Pic Velocity
- Mean Pressure Gradient (PG mean)
- AVA by Continuity Equation

DEGREE OF AORTIC STENOSIS BY PIC VELOCITY OF THE STENOTIC FLOW

Flow velocity beyond the narrowed aortic valve is studied on spectral Doppler in CW mode. The best position for the evaluation is the Apical 5 Chamber view. The flow should be as much parallel to the ultrasound beam as possible.

In the case of severe stenosis, the shape of the flow is more rounded. Mild stenosis is characterized by a peak at the beginning of systole; the flow is more triangular on the spectrogram. A late peak is characteristic of subaortic dynamic stenosis

Assessment of Aortic Stenosis by Pic Velocity:

- Mild - 2.6-2.9 m/c
- Moderate 3.0-4.0 m/s
- Severe > 4 m/s

MITRAL REGURGITATION

DEGREE OF AORTIC STENOSIS BY MEAN PRESSURE GRADIENT

The transaortic pressure gradient can assess the severity of aortic stenosis, the pressure gradient between the aorta and the left ventricle during systole.

The mean systolic pressure gradient is more consistent with cardiac catheterization data than the peak pressure gradient.

The mean gradient is calculated by averaging the pressure gradient over the entire ejection period. Calculators are embedded in echocardiographs; the operator will only trace the spectrogram.

Assessment of Aortic Stenosis by Mean Pressure Gradient:

- Mild < 20 mmHg
- Moderate 20-40 mmHg
- Severe > 40 mmHg

DEGREE OF AORTIC STENOSIS BY AORTIC VALVE AREA (AVA)

The best indicator of the severity of aortic stenosis is the area of the aortic valve opening. It is calculated from the flow continuity equation. The flow in the output tract of the left ventricle is studied in pulseless wave mode, in the aorta in continuous wave mode The calculation is based on the flow continuity equation, according to which the stroke volume of the flow in the left ventricular outflow tract is equal to the stroke volume of the transaortic flow:

$$CSA_{LVOT} = \frac{\pi D^2{}_{LVOT}}{4}$$

D - diameter of the base of the aorta. VTI_{LVOT} - integral of the linear velocity of the flow in the LV outflow tract. VTI_{AO} - integral of the linear velocity of the flow in the Aorta.

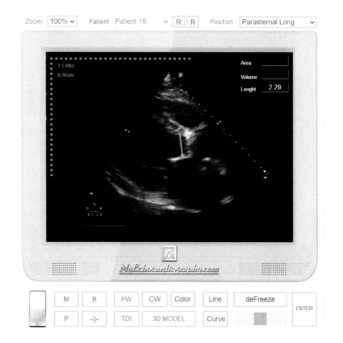

Left Parasternal View. The long axis. Measurement of the D - diameter of the base of the aorta. Simulation By Echocardiography Online Simulator MyEchocardiography.com

$$AVA = CSA_{LVOT} \times \frac{VTI_{LVOT}}{VTI_{AO}}$$

AVA - Aortic valve orifice area. CSA_{LVOT} - left ventricular outflow tract area.

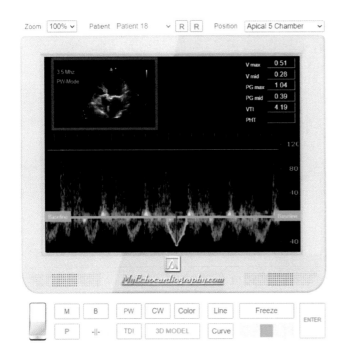

Apical 5 Chamber View. PW Doppler. Measurement of the VTI LVOT. Simulation By Echocardiography Online Simulator *MyEchocardiography.com*

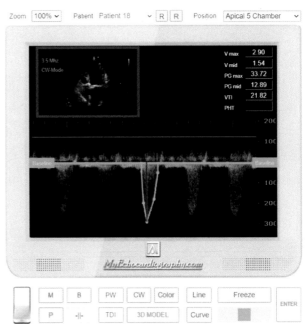

Apical 5 Chamber View. CW Doppler. Measurement of the VTI Ao. Simulation By Echocardiography Online Simulator *MyEchocardiography.com*

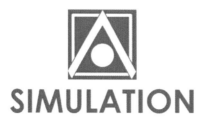

SIMULATION

AORTIC SENOSIS BY PIC VELOCITY AND MEAN PRESSURE GRADIENT

Echocardiography Online Simulator
MyEchocardiography.com

- Go to the link https://simulation.myechocardiography.com/

- Run Echocardiography Online Simulator using the **On/Off** Button

- Choose the patient 18 from the list **<<Patient>>**

- Choose **<<Apical 5 Chamber>>** from the List **<<Positions>>** or find the position with **3D Transducer**

- Click the button **<<CW>>** plase the Sample Volume in the Aorta and click.

Pic Velosity

- Click the Button **<<Calculations>>** Click Tab **<<Ao st >>** Click Radio Button **<<Pic Velocity>>**

- Click the button **<<Curve>>** and place the points around spectrogram of the Ao flow.

- Click the button **<<Enter>>**

Mean pressure gradient

- Click Radio Button **<<PG mid>>**

- Click the button **<<Curve>>** and place the points around spectrogram of the Ao flow.

- Click the button **<<Enter>>**

- Click the button << R >> to see the results.

- To change the patient, click the **On/Off** Button

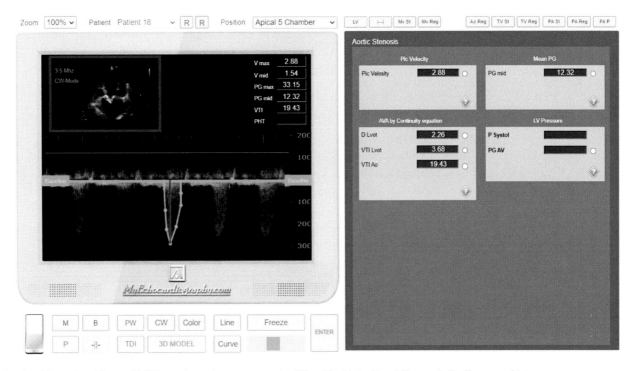

Apical 5 Chamber View. CW Doppler. Measurement of the Pic Velosity of the systolic flow and Mean pressure gradient. Aortic Stenosis. Simulation By Echocardiography Online Simulator MyEchocardiography.com

https://youtu.be/62hJZSbS1xg

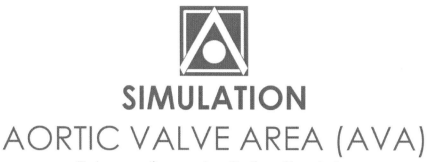

SIMULATION
AORTIC VALVE AREA (AVA)
Echocardiography Online Simulator
MyEchocardiography.com

- Go to the link https://simulation.myechocardiography.com/

- Run Echocardiography Online Simulator using the **On/Off** Button

- Choose the patient 18 from the list **<<Patient>>**

- Choose **<<Parasternal Long>>** from the List **<<Positions>>** or find the position with **3D Transducer**

- Click the Button **<<Calculations>>** Click Tab **<<Ao st >>** Click Radio Button **<<D Lvot>>** (Calculator AVA by Continuity Equation)

- Click the button **<<Line>>** and measure Left ventricular outflow tract Diameter.

- Click the button **<<Enter>>**

- Click the Radio Button **<<VTI Lvot>>** (Calculator AVA by Continuity Equation)

- Choose **<<Apical 5 Chamber>>** from the List **<<Positions>>** or find the position with 3D Transducer

- Click the button **<<PW>>** plase the Sample Volume in the Left Ventricular outflow tract and click.

- Click the button **<<Curve>>** and place the points around spectrogram of the LVOT flow.

- Click the button **<<Enter>>**

- Click the Radio Button **<<VTI Ao>>** (Calculator AVA by Continuity Equation)

- Click the button **<<CW>>** plase the Sample Volume in the Aorta and click.

- Click the button <<Curve>> and place the points around spectrogram of the Ao flow.

- Click the button **<<Enter>>**

- Click the button << R >> to see the results.

- To change the patient, click the **On/Off** Button

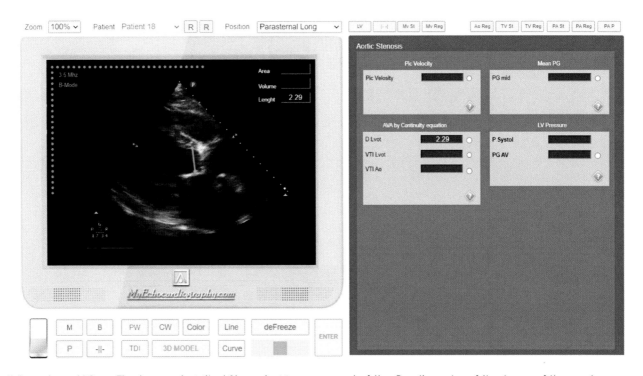

Left Parasternal View. The long axis. Mitral Stenosis. Measurement of the D - diameter of the base of the aorta.
Simulation By Echocardiography Online Simulator MyEchocardiography.com

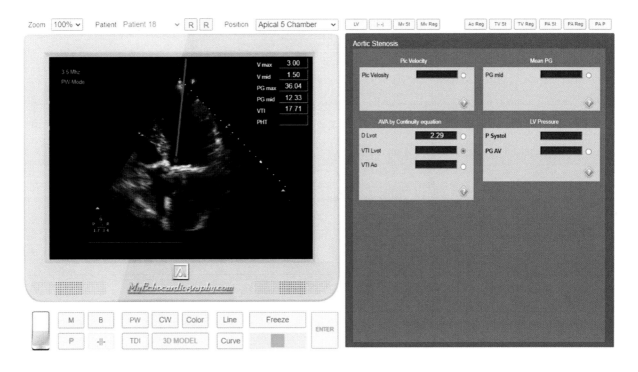

Apical 5 chamber View. Mitral Stenosis. Position of the Sample Volume for the LVOT flow. Simulation By Echocardiography Online Simulator MyEchocardiography.com

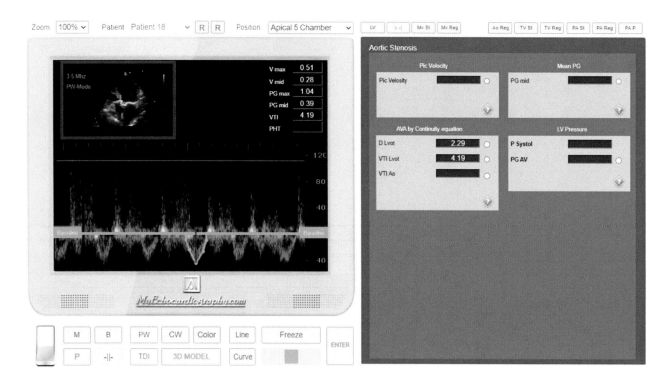

Apical 5 Chamber View. Mitral Stenosis . PW Doppler. Measurement of the VTI LVOT. Simulation By Echocardiography Online Simulator MyEchocardiography.com

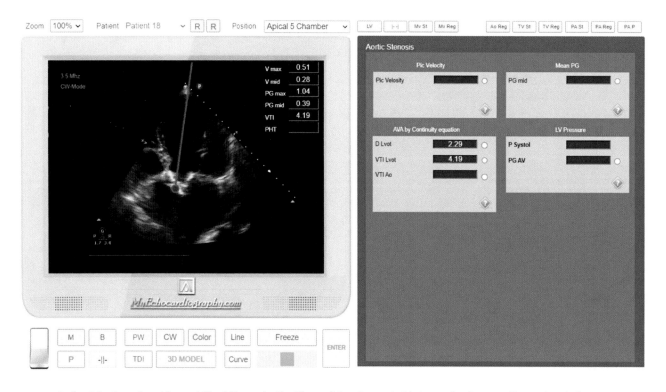

Apical 5 chamber View. Mitral Stenosis. Position of the Sample Volume for the Ao flow. Simulation By Echocardiography Online Simulator MyEchocardiography.com

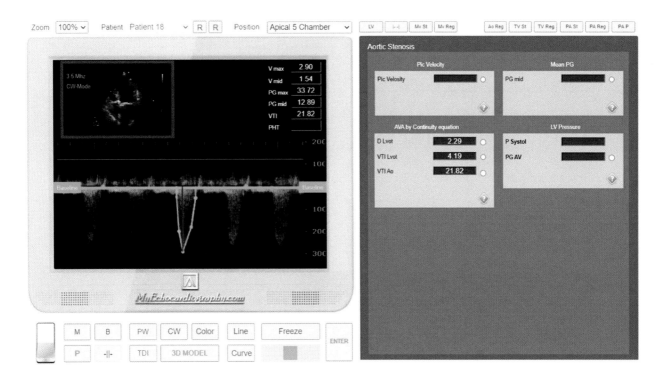

Apical 5 Chamber View. Mitral Stenosis . CW Doppler. Measurement of the VTI Ao. Simulation By Echocardiography Online Simulator MyEchocardiography.com

https://youtu.be/iZWkre-e720

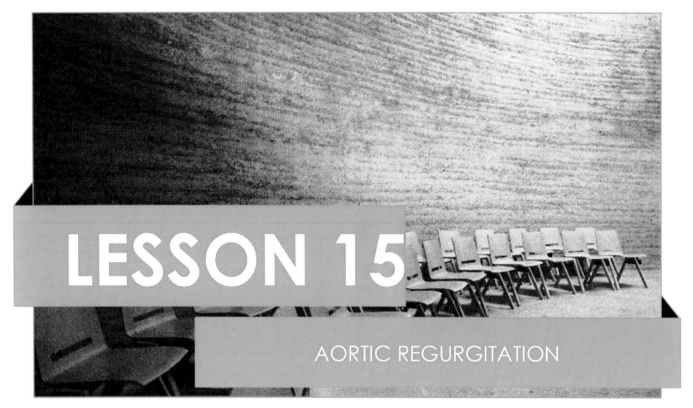

LESSON 15

AORTIC REGURGITATION

One and two-dimensional Echocardiography

The only relatively reliable specific finding can be Diastolic vibration of the anterior leaflet of the mitral valve is caused by a reversed turbulent outflow of blood from the aorta into the left ventricle (one-dimensional echocardiography).
Non-specific symptom: LV Myocardial hypertrophy and dilatation

Color Doppler

The most informative method is color, Doppler. The best positions for evaluation are the Apical 5-chamber view and the Left Parasternal View, the Long axis of the heart. Regurgitation flow is observed in the diastolic phase and returns to the left ventricle. If examining from Apical 5 Chamber View, The flow is directed towards the transducer accordingly encoded in red.

When examining from a parasternal approach the long axis of the heart, the regurgitation flow can be directed towards or away from the transducer. It depends on the orientation of the outflow tract to the ultrasound beam. If the LV outflow tract is in front of the transducer, then the regurgitation flow is directed away from the transducer and accordingly coded in blue. When positioned at the back, the flow is directed toward the transducer and coded in red.

Regurgitation size and volume depend on the severity of regurgitation.

AORTIC REGURGITATION

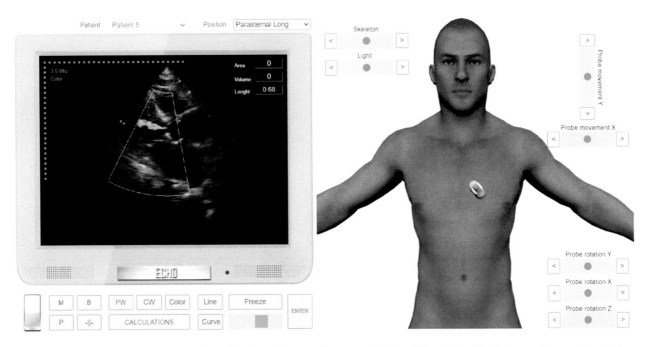

Left Parasternal View, the long axis. Color Doppler. Aortic regurgitation. Simulation By Echocardiography Online Simulator MyEchocardiography.com

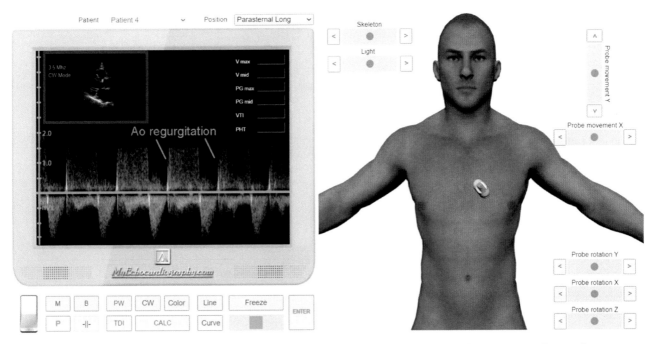

CW Doppler. Aortic regurgitation. *Simulation By Echocardiography Online Simulator MyEchocardiography.com*

Spectral Doppler (PW, CW)

The best positions for evaluation: Apical 5 Chamber View, and to find the regurgitation and determine the depth of its penetration, the sample volume is placed in the outflow tract of the left ventricle at the level of the junction of the aortic valve leaflets. After, it has to be moved at different distances from the Aortic valve (in LV).

The regurgitation flow is clearly visible on the spectrogram (both in PW and CW mode) as a characteristic spectrum above the baseline. The flow captures the entire diastole (from the aortic valve's closing to the mitral valve's opening).

Methods of assessment severity of the Aortic Regurgitation:

- PHT
- Regurgitation jet width / LVOT diameter
- Regurgitation jet area / CSA LVOT
- Vena Contracta
- Regurgitation volume and fraction (SV method)

DEGREE OF AORTIC REGURGITATION BY THE JET DECELERATION RATE (PHT)

This method is based on determining the pressure gradient half-time (PHT) between the left ventricle and the aorta.

- Align the insonation beam with the flow
- Usually best from apical windows
- In eccentric jets, it may be best from the parasternal window, helped by the color Doppler

Degree of the Aortic regurgitation by PHT:

- Mild - PHT < 500 msec
- Moderate - PHT 500-200 msec
- Severe - PHT < 200 msec

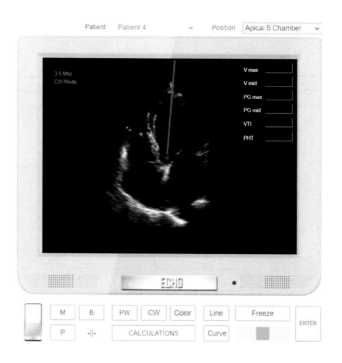

Apical 5 Chamber View. CW Doppler Control Volume in the LVOT (Left ventricular outflow tract). Simulation By Echocardiography Online
Simulator *MyEchocardiography.com*

AORTIC REGURGITATION

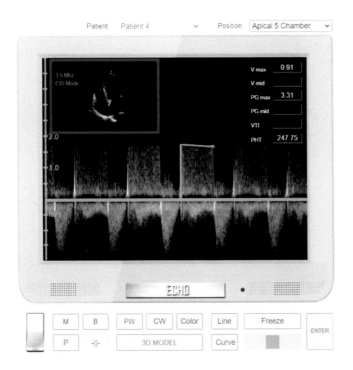

Apical 5 Chamber View. CW Doppler. Degree of Aortic Regurgitation by PHT Simulation By Echocardiography Online Simulator MyEchocardiography.com

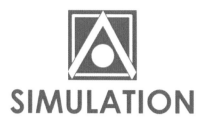

SIMULATION

DEGREE OF AORTIC REGURGITATION BY THE JET DECELERATION RATE (PHT)

Echocardiography Online Simulator
MyEchocardiography.com

- Go to the link https://simulation.myechocardiography.com/

- Run Echocardiography Online Simulator using the **On/Off** Button

- Choose the patient 4 from the list **<<Patient>>**

- Choose **<<Apical 5 chamber>>** from the List **<<Positions>>** or find the position with **3D Transducer**

- Click Button **<<Calculations>>** Click Tab **<<Ao Reg>>** Click Radio Button **<<PHT>>** (Calculator PHT).

- Click the button **<<CW>>** to move to Continuous Wave Spectral Doppler (CW).

- Place **Control Volume** in LVOT (Left ventricular outflow tract) and **click.**

- Measure PHT (See the Lesson 8).

- Click the button **<<Enter>>**

- Click the button << R >> to see the results.

- To change the patient, click the **On/Off** Button

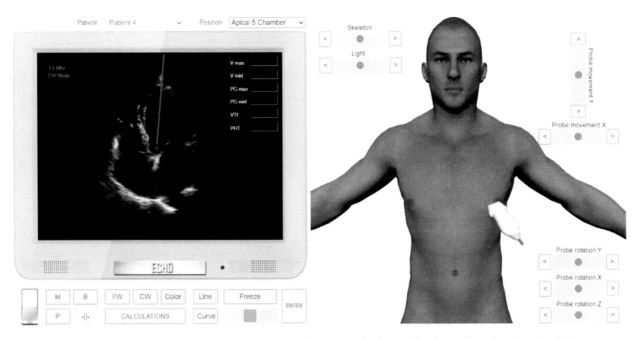

Apical 5 Chamber View. CW Doppler Control Volume in the LVOT (Left ventricular outflow tract). Simulation By Echocardiography Online Simulator MyEchocardiography.com

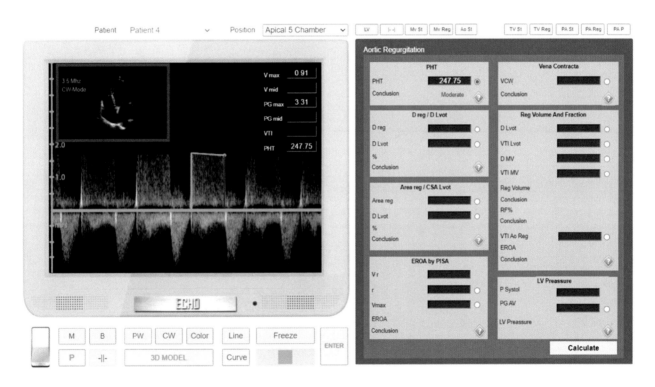

Apical 5 Chamber View. CW Doppler. Degree of Aortic Regurgitation by PHT. Simulation By Echocardiography Online Simulator MyEchocardiography.com

https://www.youtube.com/watch?v=-pGFfgl4mOs

AORTIC REGURGITATION

AORTIC REGURGITATION ASSESSMENT BY JET WIDTH / LVOT DIAMETER

The severity of aortic regurgitation can be assessed using the width of the regurgitation jet (on color Doppler) and its percentage to the diameter of the outflow tract of the left ventricle.

In the left parasternal position, the long axis of the heart, the width of the regurgitation flow is measured (1 cm distal to the aortic valve), and its percentage to the diameter of the outflow tract of the left ventricle is found.

Degree of the Aortic regurgitation by Jet width/LVOT diameter:

- Mild < 25 %
- Mild-Moderate 25-45 %
- Moderate-Severe 46-64 %
- Severe > 65 %

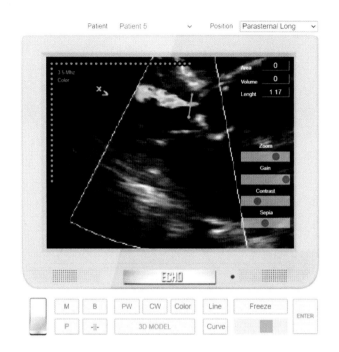

Left Parasternal View, Long axis of LV, Color Doppler. Measurement of the LVOT diameter. Simulation By Echocardiography Online Simulator _MyEchocardiography.com_

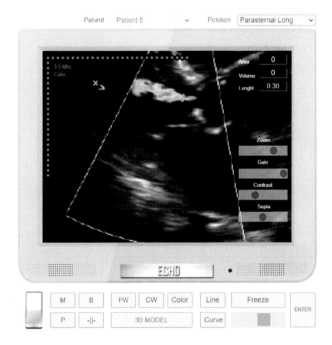

Left Parasternal View, the Long axis of LV, Color Doppler. Measurement of the regurgitation jet width. Simulation By Echocardiography Online Simulator _MyEchocardiography.com_

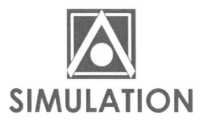

SIMULATION

AORTIC REGURGITATION ASSESSMENT BY JET WIDTH / LVOT DIAMETER

Echocardiography Online Simulator
MyEchocardiography.com

- Go to the link https://simulation.myechocardiography.com/

- Run Echocardiography Online Simulator using the **On/Off** Button

- Choose the patient 5 from the list **<<Patient>>**

- From the List **<<Positions>>** Choose **Parasternal Long** (Left Parasternal View, Long axis of LV) or find the same position with **3D Transducer**.

- Click the button **<<Color>>**

- Click the button **<<Freeze>>** to freeze image. Click the Button **<< - | | - >>** and increase zoom level. Using Slider find the best frame of Aortic regurgitation jet.

- Click Button **<<Calculations>>** Click Tab **<<Ao Reg>>** Click Radio Button **<<D reg >>** (Calculator **D reg / D Lvot**).

- Click the button **<<Line>>** measure regurgitation jet diameter in **LVOT**.

- Click the button **<<Enter>>**

- Click the button **<<Line>>** measure Diameter of LVOT (Left Ventricular Outflow Tract).

- Click the button **<<Enter>>**.

- Click the button << R >> to see the results.

- To change the patient, click the **On/Off** Button

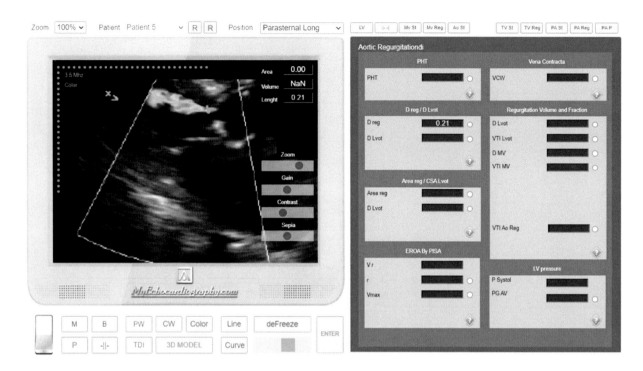

Left Parasternal View, the Long axis of LV, Color Doppler. Measurement of the regurgitation jet width. Simulation By Echocardiography Online Simulator MyEchocardiography.com

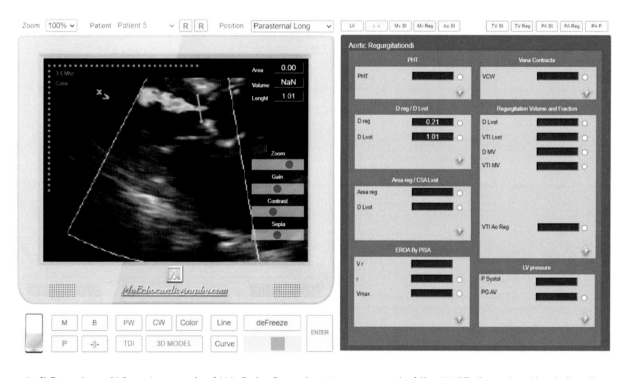

Left Parasternal View, Long axis of LV, Color Doppler. Measurement of the LVOT diameter. Simulation By Echocardiography Online Simulator MyEchocardiography.com

https://youtu.be/fry349s4YaI

AORTIC REGURGITATION

AORTIC REGURGITATION ASSESSMENT BY JET AREA/LVOT AREA

The percentage of the cross-sectional area of the regurgitation flow (CSA) to the area of the outflow tract of the left ventricle (CSA LVOT) can be used to evaluate the degree of the aortic regurgitation (In practice, these parameters are often visually assessed). In the left parasternal position, the short axis of the heart at the level of the Ao valve, the cross-sectional area of the regurgitation flow is measured planimetrically (tracing).

The formula calculates the area of the outflow tract of the left ventricle:

$$S_{LVOT} = D^2_{LVOT} \times 0.785$$

DLVOT - Diameter of the Left Ventricular Outflow tract (LVOT).

Degree of the Aortic regurgitation by Jet area/LVOT area:

- Mild < 5 %
- Mild-Moderate 5 - 20 %
- Moderate-Severe 21-59 %
- Severe > 60 %

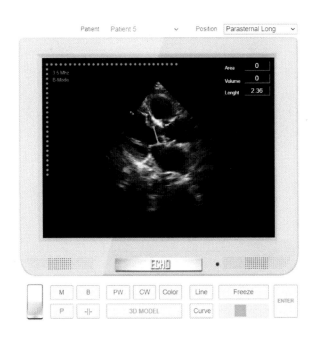

Left Parasternal View, the Long axis of LV, Measurement of the Left Ventricular Outflow Tract (LVOT) Diameter. Using this parameter, the Echocardiography calculator will measure LVOT Area. Simulation By Echocardiography Online Simulator *MyEchocardiography.com*

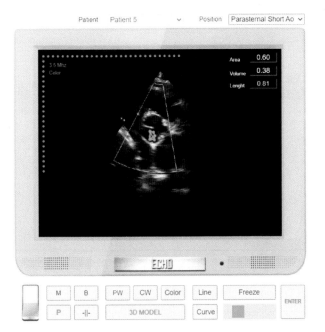

Left Parasternal View, the short axis at the level of Ao valve. Color Doppler. Measurement of the regurgitation jet area. Simulation By Echocardiography Online Simulator MyEchocardiography.com

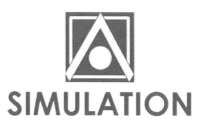

SIMULATION
AORTIC REGURGITATION ASSESSMENT BY JET AREA/LVOT AREA
Echocardiography Online Simulator
MyEchocardiography.com

- Go to the link https://simulation.myechocardiography.com/

- Run Echocardiography Online Simulator using the **On/Off** Button

- Choose the patient 5 from the list **<<Patient>>**

- From the List **<<Positions>>** Choose Parasternal Short Ao (Left Parasternal View, Short axis of Ao) or find the same position with 3D Transducer.

- Click the button **<<Color>>**

- Click the button **<<Freeze>>** to freeze image. Using Slider find the best frame of aotic regurgitation jet.

- Click Button **<<Calculations>>** Click Tab **<<Ao Reg>>** Click Radio Button **<<Area reg >>** (Calculator Area reg / CSA Lvot).

- Click the button **<<Curve>>** measure regurgitation jet area by tracing around it.

- Click the button **<<Enter>>**

- Click the button **<<Line>>** measure Diameter of LVOT (Left Ventricular Outflow Tract).

- Click the button **<<Enter>>**.

- Click the button << R >> to see the results.

- To change the patient, click the **On/Off** Button

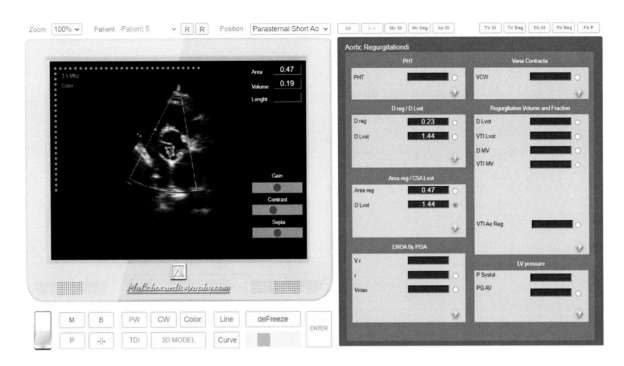

Left Parasternal View, the short axis at the level of Ao valve. Color Doppler. Measurement of the regurgitation jet area. Simulation By Echocardiography Online Simulator MyEchocardiography.com

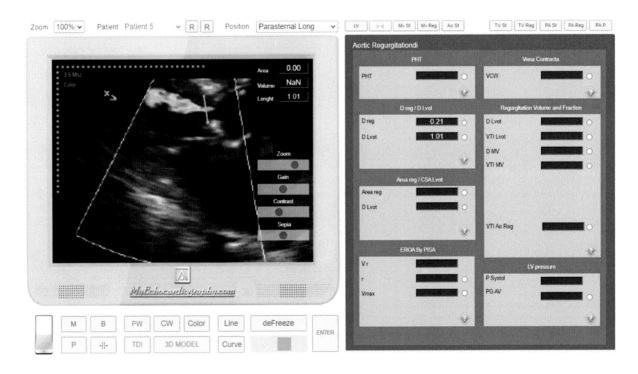

Left Parasternal View, Long axis of LV, Color Doppler. Measurement of the LVOT diameter. Simulation By Echocardiography Online Simulator MyEchocardiography.com

DEGREE OF AORTIC REGURGITATION BY VENA CONTRACTA WIDTH (VCW)

Vena contracta - this is the width of the flow at the site of its formation, the so-called neck of the regurgitation, the narrowest point of the flow, at the ends of the leaflets of the valve.

Vena contracta is best visualized and measured in a zoomed, parasternal long-axis view. Since it is the narrowest area of the jet, it is smaller than the jet width in the LVOT. It can be measured in most patients with good echocardiographic images.

Vena Contracta Width (VCW) can be used to assess the severity of regurgitation:

- Mild - Vena Contracta < 0.3 cm.
- Moderate - 0.3-0.6 cm.
- Severe - Vena Contracta > 0.6 cm.

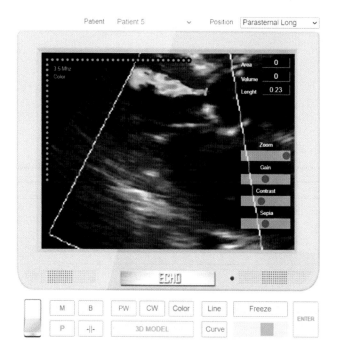

Left Parasternal View, the Long axis of LV, color Doppler, Aortic regurgitation. VCW measurement. Simulation By Echocardiography Online
Simulator *MyEchocardiography.com*

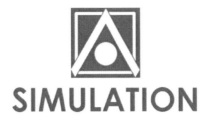

SIMULATION

DEGREE OF AORTIC REGURGITATION BY VENA CONTRACTA WIDTH (VCW)

Echocardiography Online Simulator
MyEchocardiography.com

- Go to the link https://simulation.myechocardiography.com/

- Run Echocardiography Online Simulator using the **On/Off** Button

- Choose the patient 5 from the list **<<Patient>>**

- From the List **<<Positions>>** Choose **Parasternal Long** (Left Parasternal View, Long axis of LV) or find the same position with **3D Transducer**.

- Click the button **<<Color>>**

- Click the button **<<Freeze>>** to freeze image. Click the Button **<< -| |- >>** and increase zoom level. Using Slider find the best frame of Aortic regurgitation jet.

- Click Button **<<Calculations>>**, Click Tab **<<Ao Reg>>** Click Radio Button **<<VCW >>** (Calculator **Vena Contracta**).

- Click the button **<<Line>>** measure Vena Contracta Width.

- Click the button **<<Enter>>**

- Click the button << R >> to see the results.

- To change the patient, click the **On/Off** Button

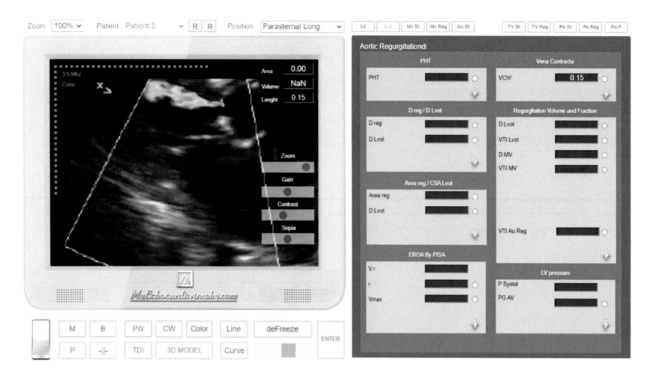

Left Parasternal View, Long axis of LV, Color Doppler. Vena Contracta Width. Simulation By Echocardiography Online Simulator MyEchocardiography.com

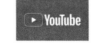

https://youtu.be/KQ1jFS12zv8

AORTIC REGURGITATION

DEGREE OF AORTIC REGURGITATION BY REGURGITATION VOLUME AND FRACTION

The volume of Aortic regurgitation is the difference between the flow in the outflow tract of the left ventricle and the transmitral flow:

$$RV = SV_{LVOT} - SV_{MV}$$

RV - regurgitation volume. SVmv - transmitral stroke Volume. SVLVOT - LVOT Stroke Volume.

To calculate the transmitral Stroke Volume (SV), it is necessary to measure the mitral annulus's D-diameter and the transmitral flow's VTI.

$$SV_{MV} = D_{MV}^2 \times 0.785 \times VTI_{MV}$$

D - diameter of the mitral annulus. VTIMV - VTI of the transmitral flow.

To calculate the stroke volume through the outflow tract of the left ventricle, it is necessary to measure the D-diameter of the LVOT and the VTI of the flow in the outflow tract of the left ventricle (LVOT).

$$SV_{LVOT} = D_{LVOT}^2 \times 0.785 \times VTI_{LVOT}$$

D - diameter of the LVOT. VTILVOT - VTI of the LVOT flow.

- LVOT diameter is measured at the annulus in systole; PW Doppler from apical views at the same site.
- Mitral annulus measured at mid diastole; PW Doppler at the annulus level in diastole.
- Total LV SV can also be measured by the difference between LV end-diastolic volume and end-systolic volume.
- LV volumes are best measured by 3D. Contrast may be needed to better trace endocardial borders. If 3D not feasible, use 2D method of disks.

Assessment of Aortic regurgitation by the regurgitation volume:

- Mild < 30 ml
- Mild-Moderate 30 – 44 ml
- Moderate-severe 45 – 59 ml
- Severe > 60 ml

Regurgitation fraction (RF%) is determined by the following formula:

$$RF(\%) = \frac{RV}{SV_{LVOT}}$$

Assessment of Aortic regurgitation by the regurgitation fraction (RF%):

- Mild < 30
- Mild-Moderate 30 - 39
- Moderate-severe 40 - 49
- Severe > 50

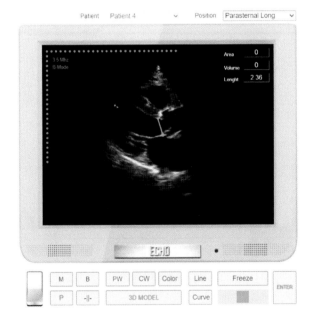

Left Parasternal View. The long axis of LV. Measurement of the Left Ventricular Outflow Tract (LVOT) diameter. Simulation By Echocardiography Online Simulator *MyEchocardiography.com*

AORTIC REGURGITATION

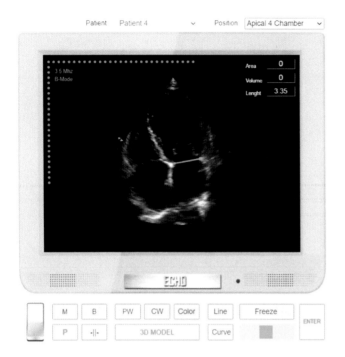

Apical 4 chamber view. Measurement of the Mitral Annulus Diameter. Simulation By Echocardiography Online Simulator MyEchocardiography.com

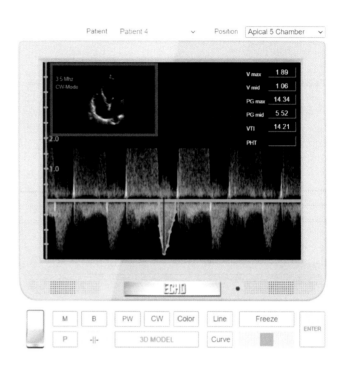

Apical 5 chamber view. CW Doppler. VTI LVOT measurement. Simulation By Echocardiography Online Simulator MyEchocardiography.com

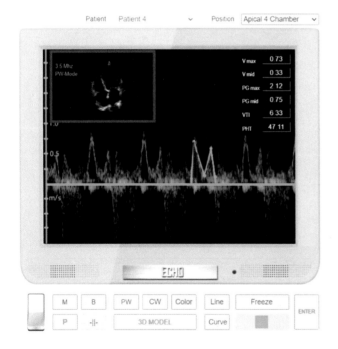

Apical 4 chamber view. PW Doppler. VTI mv measurement. Simulation By Echocardiography Online Simulator MyEchocardiography.com

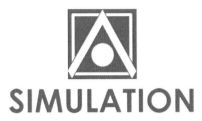

SIMULATION

DEGREE OF AORTIC REGURGITATION BY REGURGITATION VOLUME AND FRACTION

Echocardiography Online Simulator
MyEchocardiography.com

- Go to the link https://simulation.myechocardiography.com/

- Run Echocardiography Online Simulator using the **On/Off** Button

- Choose the patient 4 from the list **<<Patient>>**

- From the List **<<Positions>>** Choose **Parasternal Long** (Left Parasternal View, Long axis of LV) or find the same position with **3D Transducer.**

- Click the button **<<Freeze>>** to freeze image.

- Click Button **<<Calculations>>** Click Tab **<<Ao Reg>>** Click Radio Button **<<D Lvot>>**

- Click the button **<<Line>>** Measure linear size of **Left Ventricular Outflow Tract (LVOT).**

- Click the button **<<Enter>>**

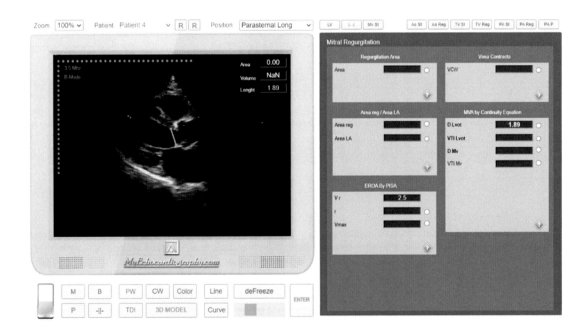

Left Parasternal View. The long axis of LV. Measurement of the Left Ventricular Outflow Tract (LVOT) diameter.
Simulation By Echocardiography Online Simulator _MyEchocardiography.com_

- From the List **<<Positions>>** Choose **Apical 4 Chamber** or find the same position with **3D Transducer**.
- Click the button **<<Freeze>>** to freeze image.
- in the Tab **<<Ao Reg>>** Click Radio Button **<<D mv>>**
- Click the button **<<Line>>** Measure **Mitral Anullus Diameter.**
- Click the button **<<Enter>>**

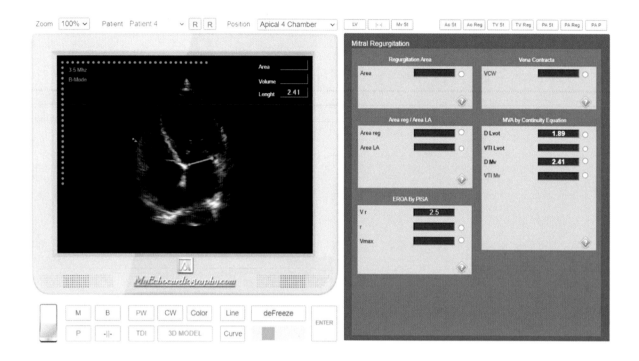

Apical 4 chamber view. Measurement of the Mitral Annulus Diameter. Simulation By Echocardiography Online Simulator MyEchocardiography.com

- In the Tab **<<Ao Reg>>** Click Radio Button **<<VTI mv>>**
- Click the button **<<PW>>** to start Pulse Wave doppler examination. Place Control Volume Beetwen Mitral Valve Leaflets and **Click**.
- Click the button **<<Curve>>** place points around spectrogram of transmitral diastolic flow.
- Click the button **<<Enter>>**

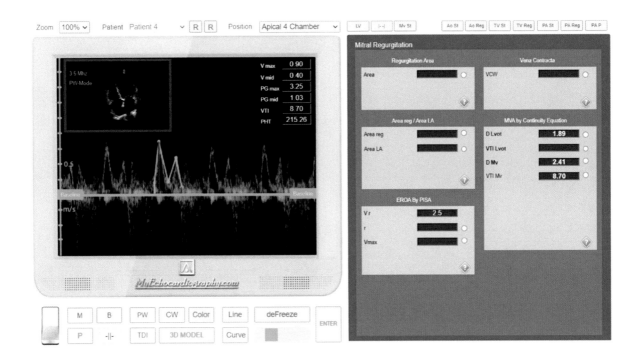

Apical 4 chamber view. PW Doppler. VTI mv measurement. Simulation By Echocardiography Online Simulator MyEchocardiography.com

- From the List **<<Positions>>** Choose **Apical 5 Chamber** or <u>find the same position with</u> **3D Transducer**.
- In the Tab **<<Ao Reg>>** Click Radio Button **<<VTI Lvot >>**
- Click the button **<<CW>>** to start Continous Wave doppler examination. Place Control Volume in LVOT and **Click**.
- Click the button **<<Curve>>** place points around spectrogram of LVOT Systolic Flow. <u>See Spectral Doppler Measurements.</u>
- Click the button **<<Enter>>**
- Click the button << **R** >> to see the results.
- To change the patient, click the **On/Off** Button

https://youtu.be/gtjxzbqugak

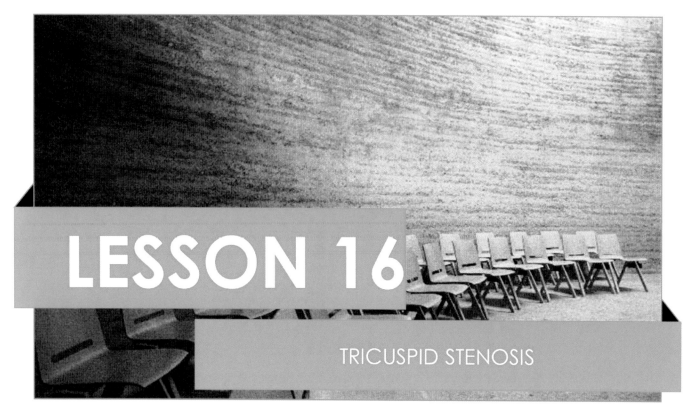

LESSON 16

TRICUSPID STENOSIS

Tricuspid stenosis is the rarest acquired heart valve disease. Its cause can be rheumatism (in such cases, as a rule, we also have mitral valve damage). It may also develop in carcinoid syndrome and endocarditis.

Two-dimensional Echocardiography

Two-dimensional echocardiography can observe calcinosis of the tricuspid valve leaflets, deformation, reduction of opening amplitude, and dilatation of the right atrium and inferior vena cava. The presence of tumors and vegetation (in the case of endocarditis) can be detected.

Spectral Doppler (PW, CW)

Spectral Doppler will reveal an increased flow rate. Still, it is worth noting that the tricuspid flow rate changes with respiratory phases, so it is necessary to average the data obtained in different respiratory cycle phases.

TRICUSPID STENOSIS

Methods of assessment severity of the Tricuspid Stenosis:

- Mean Pressure gradient
- PHT
- VTI

DEGREE OF TRICUSPID STENOSIS BY MEAN PRESSURE GRADIENT (PG mean)

- < 5 mmHg – No Significant stenosis.
- > 5 mmHg – Significant stenosis.

Degree of the Tricuspid Stenosis by PHT:

- < 190 m/s mmHg – No Significant stenosis.
- > 190 m/s mmHg – Significant stenosis.

Degree of the Tricuspid Stenosis by VTI:

- < 60 cm – No Significant stenosis.
- > 60 cm – Significant stenosis.

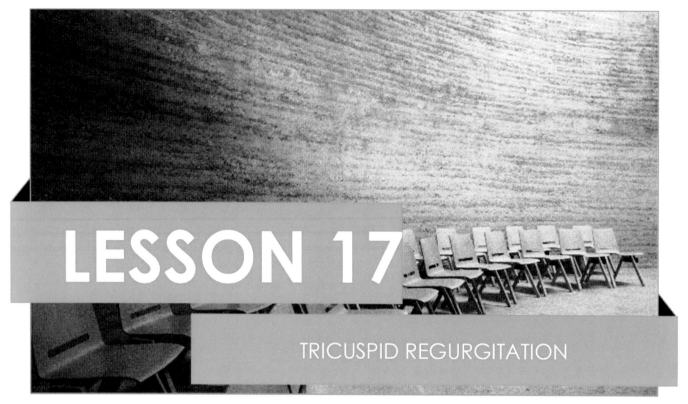

LESSON 17

Tricuspid valve insufficiency often develops secondary to right ventricular decompensation due to pulmonary hypertension. Organic damage to the valve is usually rare (endocarditis, carcinoid syndrome, Ebstein's anomaly, rheumatism). Notably, minor tricuspid regurgitation occurs in 70% of the healthy population.

Color Doppler

Direct and reliable signs can be detected only by Doppler. During color Doppler examination, we can easily see the regurgitation flow. It is coded in blue and directed towards the right atrium during the systole.

Spectral Doppler (PW, CW)

When examined by PW or CW Doppler, the regurgitation flow is directed opposite to the transducer and is located above the baseline. The flow in the hepatic veins is studied by pulsed wave Doppler, severe tricuspid regurgitation is characterized by systolic flow reversal on the spectrogram.

Spectral Doppler study of tricuspid regurgitation is also used to assess pulmonary artery pressure (systolic pressure).

LESSON CONTENT

Tricuspid Regurgitation

- Tricuspid regurgitation diagnosis.
- Degree Of Tricuspid Regurgitation By Regurgitation Area (cm2)
- Degree Of Tricuspid Regurgitation By   Pisa Radius (cm)
- Degree Of Tricuspid Regurgitation By   Hepatic Vein Flow Reversal
- Degree Of Tricuspid Regurgitation By   Density Of Regurgitation Jet

TRICUSPID REGURGITATION

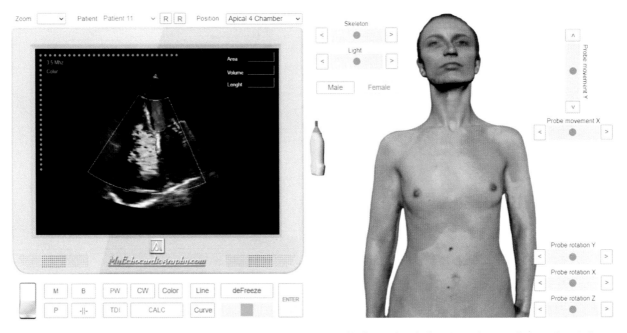

Apical Four-chamber view. Color Doppler. Tricuspid regurgitation. *Simulation By Echocardiography Online Simulator* *MyEchocardiography.com*

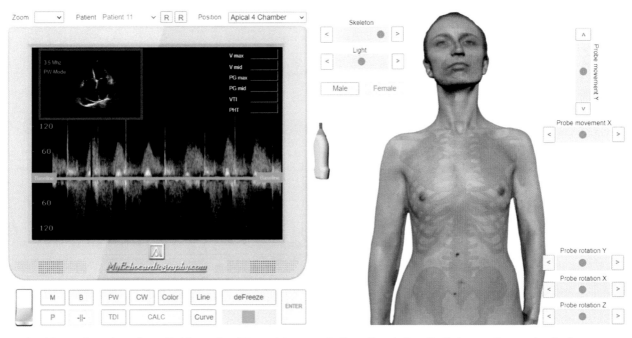

Apical Four-chamber view. PW Doppler. Tricuspid regurgitation. *Simulation By Echocardiography Online Simulator* *MyEchocardiography.com*

TRICUSPID REGURGITATION

Methods of assessment severity of the Tricuspid Regurgitation (ASE):

- Regurgitation area
- PISA
- Hepatic vein flow reversal
- Density of regurgitant jet

DEGREE OF TRICUSPID REGURGITATION BY REGURGITATION AREA (cm2)

- < 5 - mild regurgitation.
- 5 -10 - moderate regurgitation.
- > 10 - severe regurgitation.

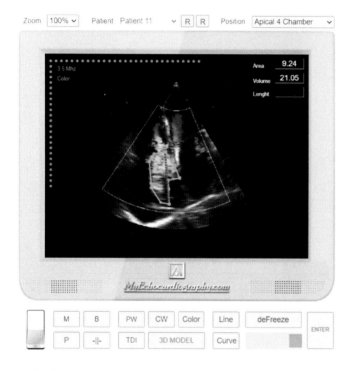

Apical Four-chamber view. Degree of Tricuspid Regurgitation by Regurgitation Area (cm2). Simulation By Echocardiography Online Simulator MyEchocardiography.com

DEGREE OF TRICUSPID REGURGITATION BY PISA radius (CM)

- < 0.5 - mild regurgitation.
- 0.5 -0.6 - moderate regurgitation.
- > 0.6 - severe regurgitation.

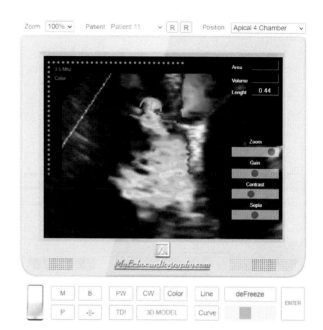

Apical Four-chamber view. Degree of Tricuspid Regurgitation by PISA. Simulation By Echocardiography Online Simulator MyEchocardiography.com

DEGREE OF TRICUSPID REGURGITATION BY HEPATIC VEIN FLOW REVERSAL

- Systolic dominance - mild regurgitation.
- Systolic blunting - moderate regurgitation.
- Systolic flow reversal - severe regurgitation.

DEGREE OF TRICUSPID REGURGITATION BY DENSITY OF REGURGITATION JET

- Faint/partial/parabolic - mild regurgitation.
- Dense, parabolic or triangular- moderate regurgitation.
- Dense, often triangular - severe regurgitation.

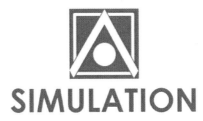

SIMULATION
DEGREE OF TRICUSPID REGURGITATION BY REGURGITATION AREA

Echocardiography Online Simulator
MyEchocardiography.com

- Go to the link https://simulation.myechocardiography.com/
- Run Echocardiography Online Simulator using the **On/Off** Button
- Choose the patient 11 from the list **<<Patient>>** (or other patient with TR)
- Choose **<<Apical 4 chamber>>** from the List **<<Positions>>** or find the position with **3D Transducer**
- Click the Button <<**Color**>>
- Click the Button <<**Freeze**>> and Using Slider find The frame where the size of the regurgitation flow is maximum.
- Click the Button **<<Calculations>>** Click Tab **<<TV Reg>>** Click Radio Button **<< Reg Area>>** (Regurgitation Area).
- Click the button **<<Curve>>** and trace around regurgitation Jet.
- Click the button **<<Enter>>**
- Click the button << **R** >> to see the results.
- To change the patient, click the **On/Off** Button

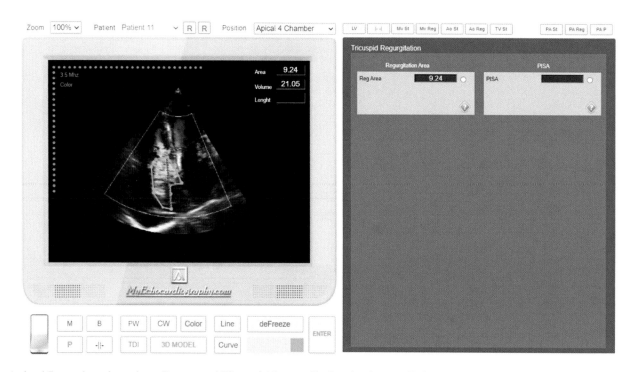

Apical Four-chamber view. Degree of Tricuspid Regurgitation by Regurgitation Area (cm2). Simulation By Echocardiography Online Simulator MyEchocardiography.com

https://youtu.be/TSeBHdjS4iw

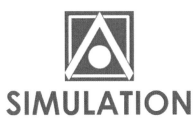

SIMULATION
DEGREE OF TRICUSPID REGURGITATION BY PISA

Echocardiography Online Simulator
MyEchocardiography.com

- Go to the link https://simulation.myechocardiography.com/
- Run Echocardiography Online Simulator using the **On/Off** Button
- Choose the patient 11 from the list **<<Patient>>** (or other patient with TR)
- Choose **<<Apical 4 chamber>>** from the List **<<Positions>>** or find the position with **3D Transducer**
- Click the Button <<**Color**>>
- Click the button **<<Freeze>>** to freeze image. Click the Button **<< - | | - >>** and increase zoom level. Using Slider find the best frame for PISA measurement. The Nyquist Limit is set to 2.5.
- Click Button **<<Calculations>>** Click Tab **<<TV Reg>>** Click Radio Button **<<PISA>>**
- Click the button **<<Line>>** measure radius of the PISA.
- Click the button **<<Enter>>**
- Click the button << **R** >> to see the results.
- To change the patient, click the **On/Off** Button

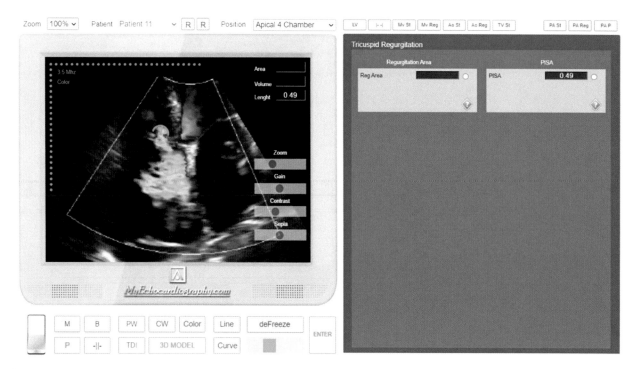

Apical Four-chamber view. Degree of Tricuspid Regurgitation by PISA. Simulation By Echocardiography Online Simulator MyEchocardiography.com

https://youtu.be/M-7p5mNj0QE

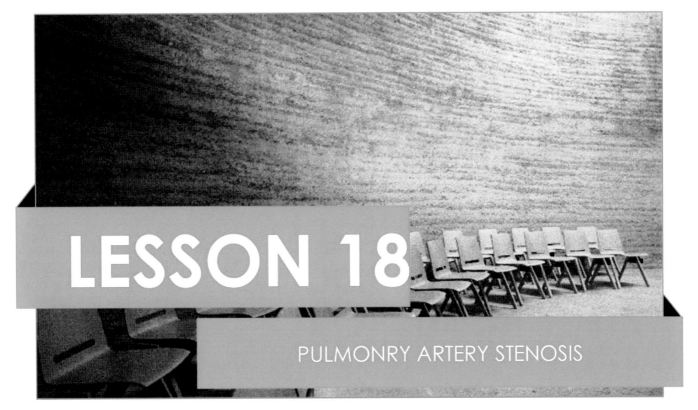

Pulmonary artery orifice stenosis is one of the most common congenital malformations. More often, it is isolated, but sometimes it is accompanied by acquired infravalvular stenosis (supravalvular stenosis can be the result of hypertrophy of the infundibular part of the ventricular septum), congenital infravalvular stenosis, pulmonary artery branch stenosis, and atrial septal defects.

A stenotic pulmonary valve can be tricuspid, bicuspid, unicuspid, or dysplastic. Pulmonary artery stenosis is included in the combination of the tetrad of Fallot. Acquired pulmonary stenosis is rare.

Two-dimensional Echocardiography

Two-dimensional echocardiography reveals the leaflets' systolic rounding, thickening, and movement in one direction. Sometimes post-stenotic expansion of the pulmonary trunk, reduction of its systolic pulsation, and hypertrophy of the right ventricle.

Spectral Doppler (PW, CW)

Spectral Doppler will reveal an increased flow rate.

LESSON CONTENT

Pulmonary Valve Stenosis

- Pulmonary Valve stenosis diagnosis.
- Degree of the pulmonary Valve stenosis by stenotic flow velocity:
- Degree of the Pulmonary Valve Stenosis by systolic pressure gradient (PG max):

Methods of assessment severity of the Pulmonary Valve Stenosis:

- Flow Velocity
- systolic pressure gradient (PG max)

DEGREE OF THE PULMONARY VALVE STENOSIS BY SYSTOLIC PRESSURE GRADIENT (PG MAX):

- Mild < 36 mmHg
- Moderate 36 – 64 m/s
- Severe > 64 m/s

DEGREE OF THE PULMONARY VALVE STENOSIS BY STENOTIC FLOW VELOCITY:

- Mild < 3 m/s
- Moderate 3 – 4 m/s
- Severe > 4 m/s

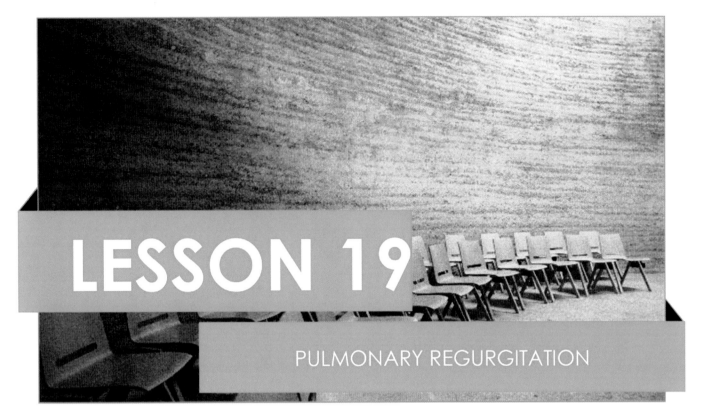

LESSON 19

PULMONARY REGURGITATION

Small functional regurgitation of the pulmonary valve occurs in approximately 78% of the healthy population. It is not heard by auscultation, but it is detected by Doppler examination and allows us to determine the end-diastolic pressure in the pulmonary artery.

Color Doppler

Color Doppler examination reveals diastolic flow in the right ventricle. When examining with the color Doppler, in the parasternal position, on the heart's short axis, the regurgitation flow is coded in red color.

Spectral Doppler (PW, CW)

Pulmonary regurgitation can be detected using Spectral Doppler examination by placing a control volume under the valve leaflets in the right ventricular outflow tract (parasternal position, short axis).

The regurgitation flow is directed to the transducer side and therefore registers above the baseline on the spectrogram.

PULMONARY REGURGITATION

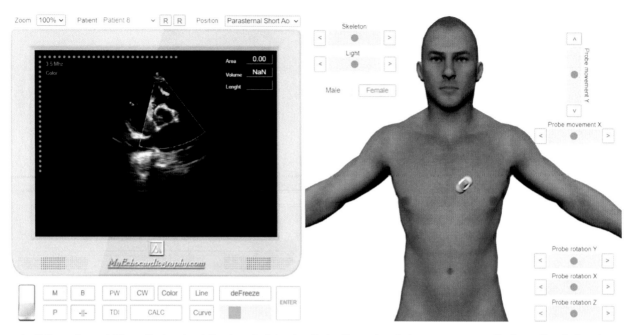

Left Parasternal View. Sort axis at the level of Aorta. Color Doppler. Pulmonary regurgitation. Simulation By Echocardiography Online Simulator MyEchocardiography.com

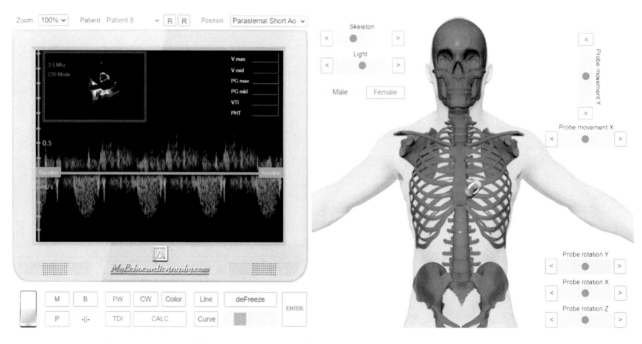

Left Parasternal View. Sort axis at the level of Aorta. Color Doppler. Pulmonary regurgitation. Simulation By Echocardiography Online Simulator MyEchocardiography.com

PULMONARY REGURGITATION

Methods of assessment severity of the Pulmonary Regurgitation (ASE):

- Regurgitation jet size
- Density of regurgitation jet

DEGREE OF TPULMONARY REGURGITATION BY DENSITY OF REGURGITATION JET (CW)

- Soft - mild regurgitation.
- Dense - moderate regurgitation.
- Dense; early termination of diastolic
- Flow - severe regurgitation.

DEGREE OF PULMONARY REGURGITATION BY REGURGITATION JET SIZE (mm)

- < 10 - mild regurgitation.
- > 10 - severe regurgitation.

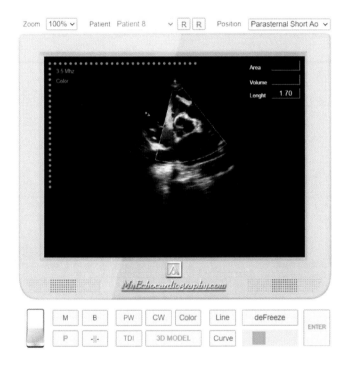

Left Parasternal View. Sort axis at the level of Aorta.
Degree of Pulmonary Regurgitation by Regurgitation jet
size. Simulation By Echocardiography Online
Simulator MyEchocardiography.com

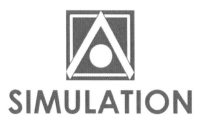

SIMULATION

DEGREE OF PULMONARY REGURGITATION BY REGURGITATION JET SIZE

Echocardiography Online Simulator
MyEchocardiography.com

- Go to the link https://simulation.myechocardiography.com/
- Run Echocardiography Online Simulator using the **On/Off** Button
- Choose the patient 8 from the list **<<Patient>>** (or other patient with PR)
- Choose **<<Parasternal Short Ao>>** from the List **<<Positions>>** or find the position with **3D Transducer**
- Click the Button <<**Color**>>
- Click the Button <<**Freeze**>> and Using Slider find The frame where the size of the regurgitation flow is maximum.
- Click the Button **<<Calculations>>** Click Tab **<<PA Reg>>** Click Radio Button **<< Jet Size>>** (Regurgitation Jet Size).
- Click the button **<<Line>>** and measure the Jet size.
- Click the button **<<Enter>>**
- Click the button << R >> to see the results.
- To change the patient, click the **On/Off** Button

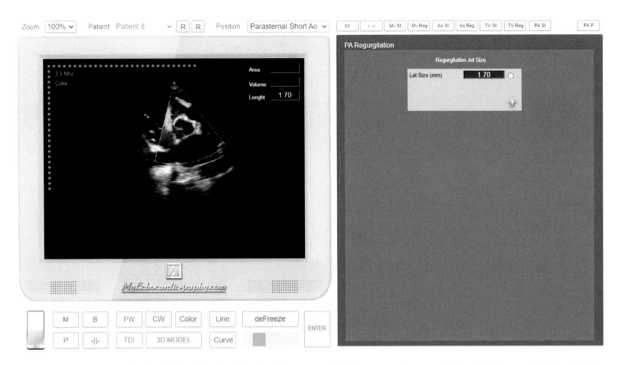

Left Parasternal View. Sort axis at the level of Aorta. Degree of Pulmonary Regurgitation by Regurgitation jet size.
Simulation By Echocardiography Online Simulator MyEchocardiography.com

https://youtu.be/dJMCHQ54HV4

CONGENITAL HEART DEFECTS IN ADULTS

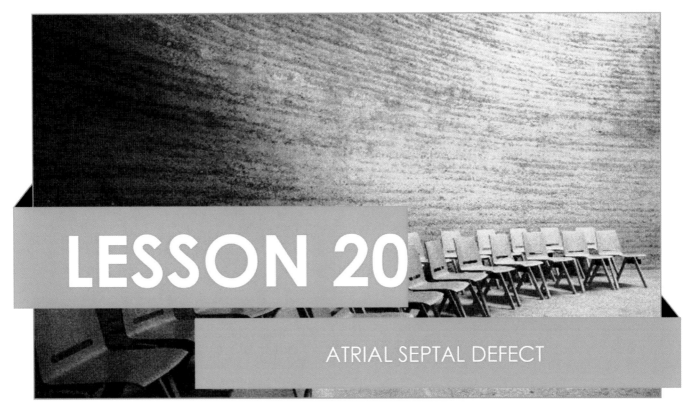

LESSON 20

ATRIAL SEPTAL DEFECT

The reason for the transfer of blood between the chambers of the heart can be:

- Atrial septal defect.
- Ventricular septal defect.
- Valsalva sinus aneurysm damage.
- Open Ductus arteriosus.
- Coronary fistulas.

Among congenital heart defects, in terms of prevalence, atrial septal defect takes second place (after bicuspid aortic valve).

Atrial septal defect is classified according to its location.

LESSON CONTENT

Atrial Septal Defect

- Echocardiography Evidense of Atrial Septal Defect.
- Two-dimensional echocardiography
- Color Doppler
- Spectral Doppler

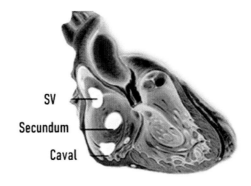

SV
Secundum
Caval

SV - Sinus Venosus

ATRIAL SEPTAL DEFECT

Two-dimensional echocardiography

With a two-dimensional study, a direct echocardiographic sign of an atrial septal defect is the finding of a break in the echo signal from the atrial septum (parasternal and subcostal position). It should be noted that in the apical four-chamber position, even in the absence of an atrial septal defect, a break in the echo signal can be detected.

Indirect signs are dilatation of the right atrium and paradoxical movement of the interventricular septum (signs of diastolic volume overload of the right heart).

Color Doppler

In color Doppler examination, if there is blood flow from left to right, the flow is coded in red. If from right to left - in blue.

Spectral Doppler

When examining in pulse wave mode, a control volume is placed in front of the suspected defect. It is possible to determine the presence and direction of the shunt.

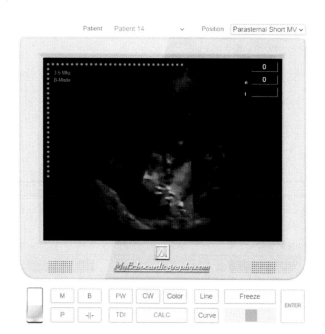

Apical Four Chamber View. Color Doppler. Atrial Septal Defect. Flow from the left to the right. Simulation By Echocardiography Online Simulator MyEchocardiography.com

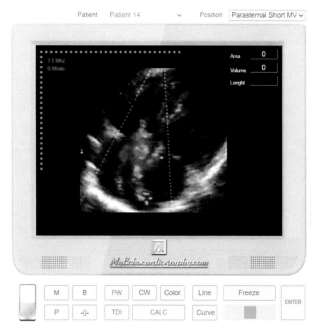

Apical Four Chamber View. Color Doppler. Atrial Septal Defect. Flow from the left to the right. Simulation By Echocardiography Online Simulator MyEchocardiography.com

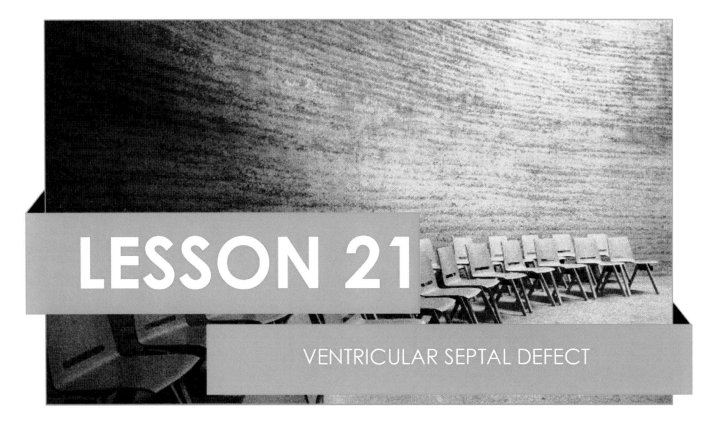

LESSON 21

VENTRICULAR SEPTAL DEFECT

The ventricular septal defect may be isolated or included in another combined malformation.

Anatomically, the interventricular septum consists of membranous and muscular parts. The membranous part is located under the aortic valve, so it is also called subaortic.

Most often (in 80% of cases) the defect is located on the membranous septum and extends to the surrounding muscle areas.

Two-dimensional echocardiography

Significant size defect can be detected by two-dimensional echocardiography. Sometimes it is possible to see the breaking of the echo signal of the interventricular septum.

Color Doppler

In color Doppler examination, if there is blood flow from left to right, the flow is coded in red. If from right to left - in blue.

Blood pumping in different directions during different phases of the cardiac cycle may indicate Eisenmenger syndrome.

LESSON CONTENT

Ventricular Septal Defect

- Echocardiography Evidense of Atrial Septal Defect.
- Two-dimensional echocardiography
- Color Doppler
- Spectral Doppler

Spectral Doppler

When examining in pulse wave mode, a control volume is placed in front of the suspected defect. It is possible to determine the presence and direction of the shunt.

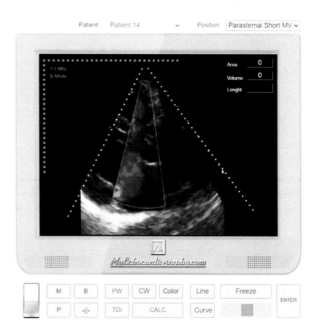

Left Parasternal View, Long axis. Color Doppler. Ventricular Septal Defect. *Simulation By Echocardiography Online Simulator MyEchocardiography.com*

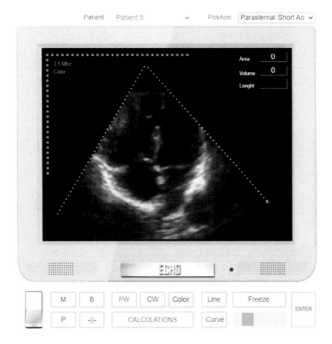

Apical Four Chamber View. B-mode. Ventricular Septal Defect. *Simulation By Echocardiography Online Simulator MyEchocardiography.com*

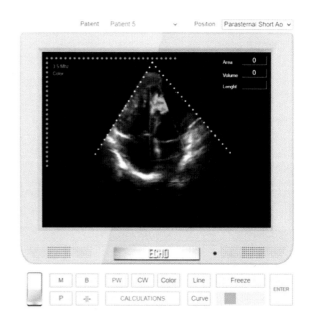

Apical Four Chamber View. Color Doppler. Ventricular Septal Defect. *Simulation By Echocardiography Online Simulator MyEchocardiography.com*

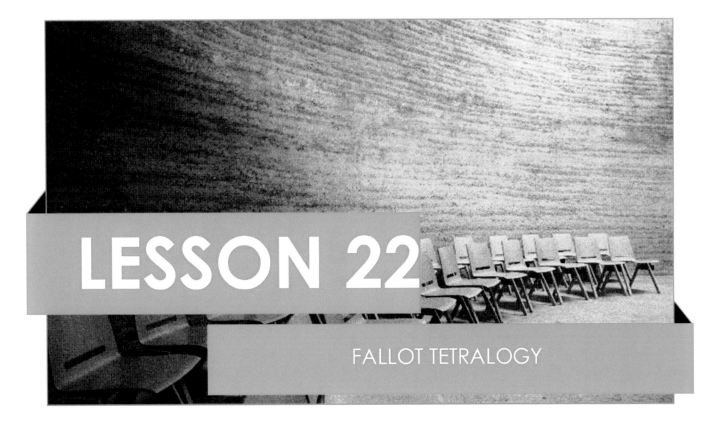

LESSON 22

FALLOT TETRALOGY

In 1888, Fallot described a malformation that included four different anomalies: a large septal defect, pulmonary artery stenosis, aortic dextraposition, and right ventricular hypertrophy. It was found that, in addition to this, 15% of patients have an atrial septal defect, 25% have a right-sided aortic arch, and 5-9% have an anterior-descending coronary artery coming out of the right coronary artery.

Two-dimensional Echocardiography

Two-dimensional echocardiographic examination, in the left parasternal position, on the long axis, will reveal a significant defect of the interventricular septum and the aorta sitting on the interventricular septum.

In the parasternal position, on the short axis, we can observe the trunk of the lung. Stenosis of the pulmonary artery can be: subvalvular, valvular and supravalvular.

Color Doppler

The flow through the defect is usually directed from right to left and can be examined by the Color Doppler.

FALLOT TETRALOGY

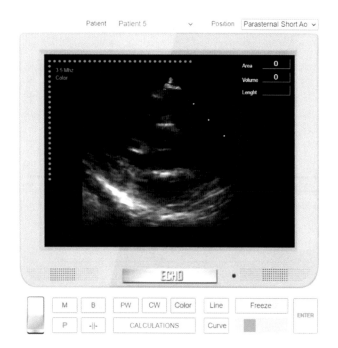

Left Parasternal View, Long axis. fallot tetralogy.
Simulation By Echocardiography Online
Simulator MyEchocardiography.com

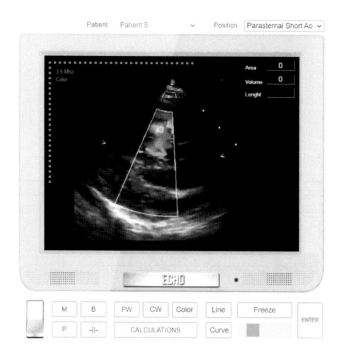

Left Parasternal View, Long axis. Color Doppler.
fallot tetralogy. Simulation By Echocardiography
Online Simulator MyEchocardiography.com

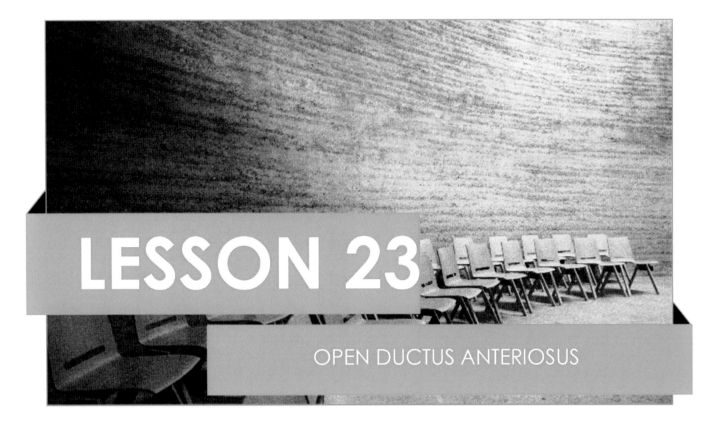

LESSON 23

OPEN DUCTUS ANTERIOSUS

Open ductus arteriosus accounts for 2% of all congenital malformations. It mainly exists independently, but sometimes it is in combination with other malformations: ventricular septal defect, coarctation of the aorta.

Two-dimensional Echocardiography

Open ductus arteriosus can be seen in children (rarely in adults) by two-dimensional echocardiography. The examination is performed from a suprasternal or parasternal approach on the short axis of the aorta.

The bifurcation of the pulmonary trunk becomes a **"trifurcation."**

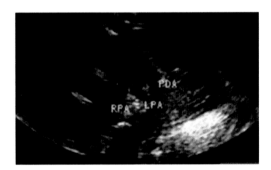

Two-dimensional echocardiography, parasternal position, the short axis of the heart. Patient with patent ductus arteriosus. The transformation of the bifurcation of the pulmonary trunk into a "trifurcation" is noted.

LESSON CONTENT

Open ductus arteriosus
- Echocardiography Evidense of Open ductus arteriosus.
- Two-dimensional echocardiography
- Color Doppler

Color Doppler

If there is left-to-right flow, color Doppler examination shows high-velocity flow starting from the aortic arch and extending along the lateral wall of the pulmonary trunk in the direction of the pulmonary artery valve. It appears in the middle or beginning of systole, reaches its maximum speed at the beginning of diastole, and almost disappears at the end.

In high pulmonary resistance, when the direction of flow changes, a Doppler examination of the descending aorta may reveal a left-right shunt of blood below the ductus arteriosus.

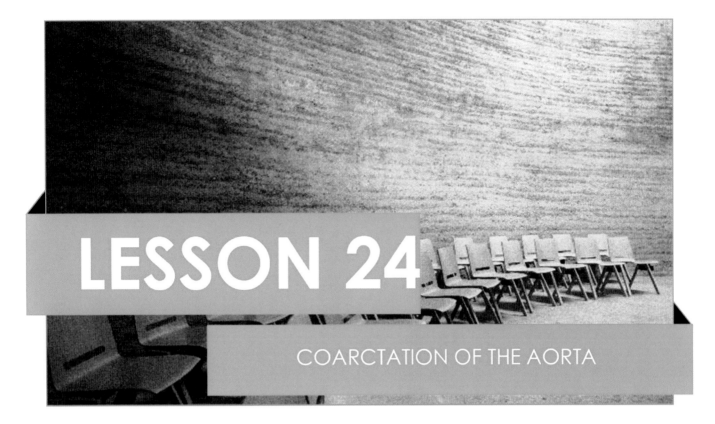

LESSON 24

COARCTATION OF THE AORTA

The coarctation is typically located below the exit site of the left clavicle. It is rarely found on the descending aorta, even more rarely on the abdominal aorta.

The aortic narrowing can be seen by transthoracic two-dimensional examination in children but rarely in adults. Post-stenotic dilatation of the aorta is almost always observed.

Half of the patients have a bicuspid aortic valve. Sometimes coarctation of the aorta is accompanied by subaortic stenosis, congenital defects of the mitral valve, and open ductus arteriosus.

Transesophageal echocardiography has a great advantage over transthoracic echocardiography in the diagnosis of coarctation of the aorta. It is possible to accurately determine the location of the coarctation and the degree of narrowing.

Two-dimensional Echocardiography

Open ductus arteriosus can be seen in children (rarely in adults) by two-dimensional echocardiography. The examination is performed from a suprasternal or parasternal approach on the short axis of the aorta.

The bifurcation of the pulmonary trunk becomes a **"trifurcation."**

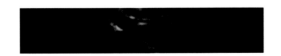

LESSON CONTENT

Coarctation of the aorta
- Echocardiography Evidense of Open Coarctation of the aorta.
- Two-dimensional echocardiography
- Color Doppler

Spectral Doppler (PW, CW)

PW examination of the descending aorta allows us to detect an increase in the flow rate. With the CW Doppler, we can measure its velocity and pressure gradient.

Color Doppler

Color Doppler examination reveals turbulent flow distal to the narrowing.

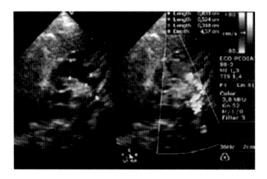

Two-dimensional echocardiography, suprasternal approach. A patient with coarctation of the aorta. Color Doppler image on the right shows turbulent flow distal to the coarctation.

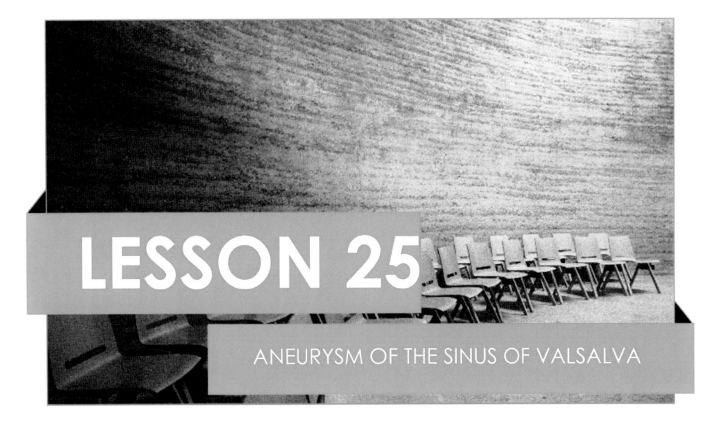

LESSON 25

ANEURYSM OF THE SINUS OF VALSALVA

Congenital aneurysm of the sinus of Valsalva is a thinning of its media in the area of the transition to the fibrous, valvular annulus.

Small aneurysms, which appear as finger-like protrusions occur more often in the right and non-coronary sinuses.

Most often, an aneurysm is detected when it is damaged. Mostly at the age of 10-30.

Two-dimensional Echocardiography

With the two-dimensional examination, it is possible to visualize the aneurysm of the sinus of Valsalva.

Color Doppler

With the Color Doppler aneurism damage can be found.

ANEURYSM OF THE SINUS OF VALSALVA

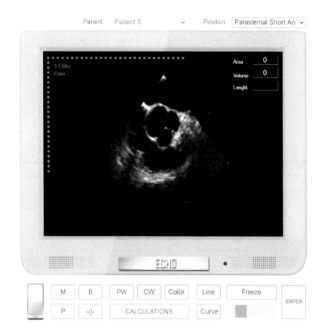

Left Parasternal View, Short axis at the level of the Aorta. Aneurysm of the sinus of Valsalva. *Simulation By Echocardiography Online Simulator* *MyEchocardiography.com*

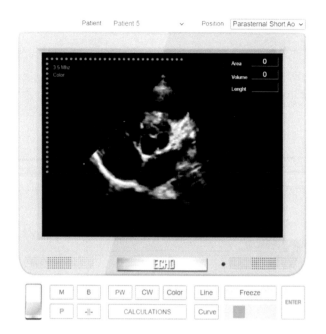

Left Parasternal View, Short axis at the level of the Aorta. Aneurysm of the sinus of Valsalva. A patient with a four-Leaflet aortic valve. *Simulation By Echocardiography Online Simulator* *MyEchocardiography.com*

INFECTIVE ENDOCARDITIS

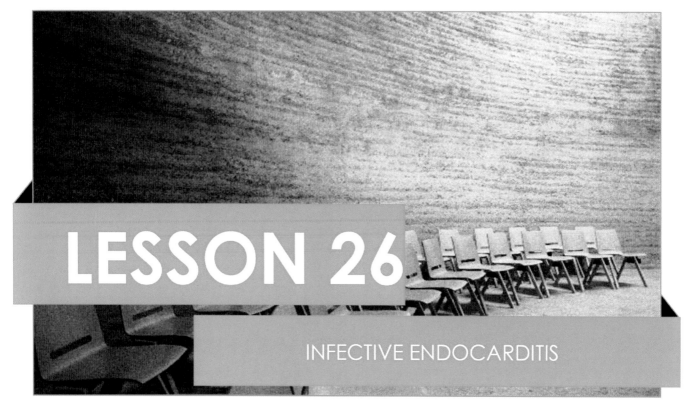

LESSON 26

INFECTIVE ENDOCARDITIS

Infective endocarditis is a severe inflammation of the endocardium, mainly due to damage to the valves.

Damage to the heart is manifested by the formation of vegetations, violation of the integrity of the chambers, and damage to the endocardium of subvalvular structures.
Nonvalvular vegetations can be located on the interventricular and atrial septum, papillary muscles, and atrium.
The mitral and aortic valves are most often damaged rarely the tricuspid and pulmonary artery valves.
Echocardiography can detect vegetation, its localization, diameter, complications and observe the process in dynamics.

In 1994, Duke University Medical Center proposed a diagnostic scheme for infective endocarditis called the Duke criteria.

Two-dimensional echocardiography

Two-dimensional echocardiography plays a central role in diagnosing and monitoring infective endocarditis. The first sign is the discovery of masses or vegetations in the myocardium, annular abscesses, and newly developed valvular regurgitation.

Transthoracic (TTE) examination (at optimal image quality) can visualize vegetation 3-5 mm in diameter; smaller vegetations are detected by transesophageal (TEE) echocardiography.

INFECTIVE ENDOCARDITIS

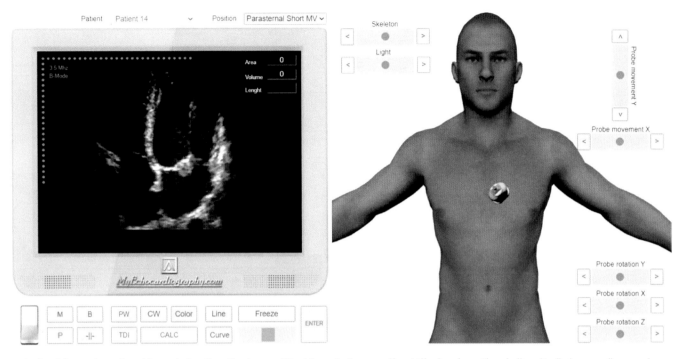

Apical four chamber View. Infective Endocarditis. Vegetation on the Mitral valve. Simulation By Echocardiography Online Simulator MyEchocardiography.com

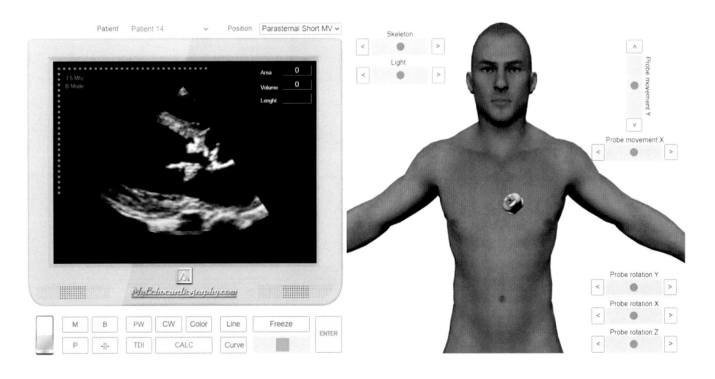

Left Parasternal View. Long axis. Vegetation on Mitral and the Aortic valve. Simulation By Echocardiography Online Simulator MyEchocardiography.com

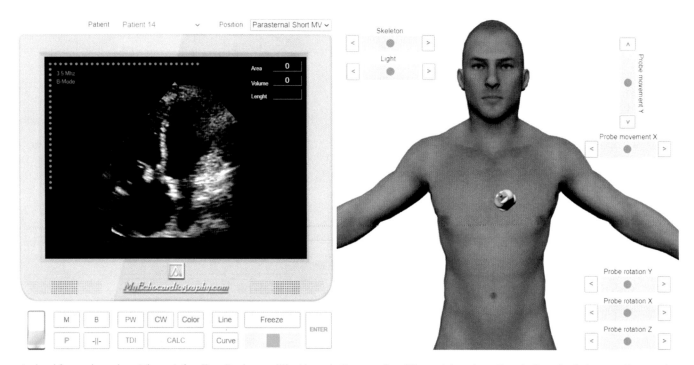

Apical four chamber View. Infective Endocarditis. Vegetation on the Tricuspid valve. Simulation By Echocardiography Online Simulator MyEchocardiography.com

PERICARDIAL EFFUSION

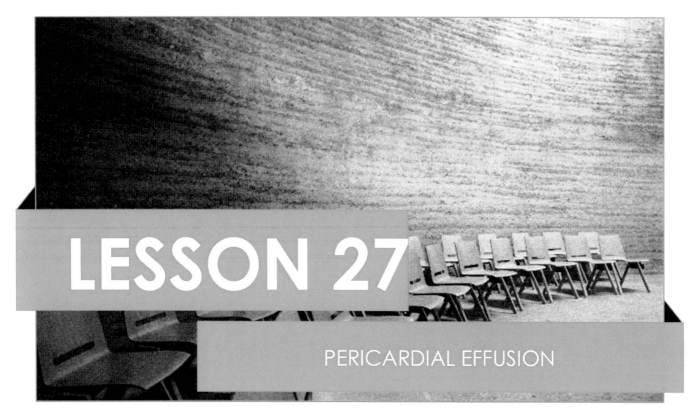

LESSON 27

PERICARDIAL EFFUSION

In the case of Pericardial Effusion, the volume of the liquid is more significant than its physiological value (Trivial 50-80 ml). Echocardiography is the initial procedure of choice to detect the presence of a Pericardial Effusion because it can be performed with minimal delay and has an accuracy of nearly 100%.

One-Dimensional Echocardiography (M-mode)

One-Dimensional examination shows the persistence of an echo-free space between the epicardium and parietal pericardium throughout the cardiac cycle. Separation of the two layers seen only in systole represents an ordinary or clinically insignificant amount of pericardial fluid (trivial PE). In contrast, a separation in systole and diastole is associated with effusions of >50 mL (small PE). M-modal examination is best done from a parasternal approach.

Usually, the parietal layer of the pericardium is one of the brightest structures of the heart. If the signal gain is maximally reduced, only the parietal pericardium will remain on the screen because it reflects the ultrasonic beam more than other structures of the heart.
Usually, the layers of the pericardium move in parallel. With exudative pericarditis, the parallel movement disappears. We see the separation of the layers and the formation of an echo-negative space between them. Diagnostic value has diastolic separation of the layers. Movement of the parietal pericardium is reduced or completely disappears.

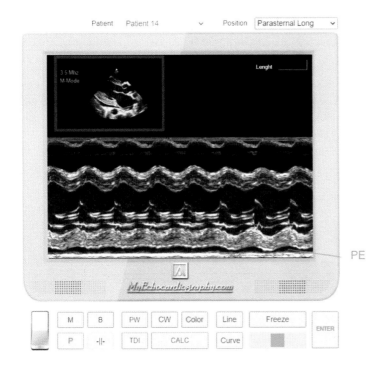

M-modal examination. Left Parasternal View, Long axis of the Heart. Pericardial effusion. Simulation By Echocardiography Online Simulator MyEchocardiography.com

Two-Dimensional Echocardiography (B-mode)

The primary diagnostic method - is Two-Dimensional Echocardiography. It helps to identify pathological fluid and determine the volume and its effect on hemodynamics.

Studies are mainly carried out from the left Parasternal approach (long and short axis of the heart) from the Apical four-chamber position and the Subcostal approach.

When examined from the Left Parasternal approach, the long-axis fluid is most often located behind the posterior wall of the left ventricle. Four pulmonary veins are attached to the left atrium; the layers of the pericardium of this area are fused and do not separate even with the accumulation of a large volume of fluid. Therefore, fluid accumulation is rare in this area, but sometimes it is observed.

When examined from the Apical Four-chamber position, the fluid is mainly behind the right atrium wall and right ventricle.

2D echocardiography shows the persistence of echo-free space between the layers of the pericardium. If the fluid accumulation age is one month, then it is transparent; if more than 1 month, fibrin strands are formed. The more pronounced fibrin, the long process we are dealing with.

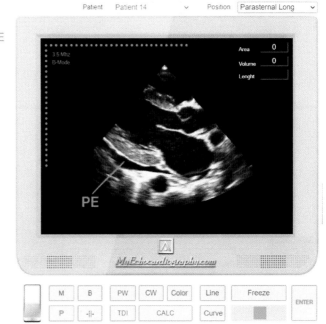

Left Parasternal View, Long axis of the Heart. Pericardial effusion. Simulation By Echocardiography Online Simulator MyEchocardiography.com

Determining the volume of Pericardial Effusion

- Trivial (seen only in systole).
- 5-10 mm separation - small (100-250 ml liquid).
- 10-20 mm separation - moderate (250-500 ml liquid).
- >20 mm separation - large (more than 500 ml of liquid).
- >25 mm - very large

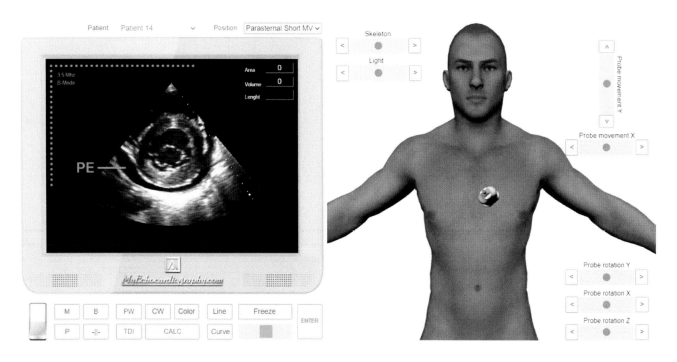

Left Parasternal View, Short axis at the level of the mitral valve. Pericardial effusion. Simulation By Echocardiography Online Simulator MyEchocardiography.com

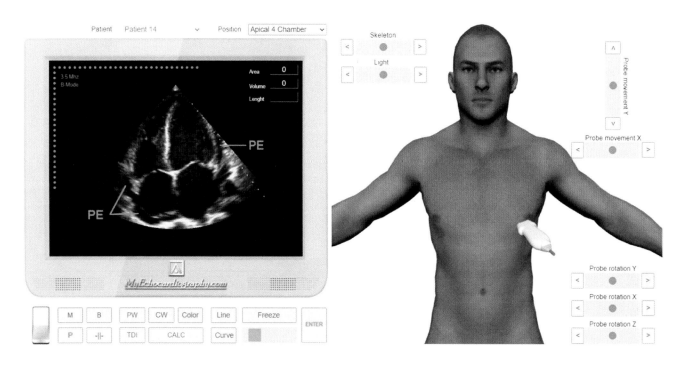

Apical 4 Chamber View. Pericardial effusion. Simulation By Echocardiography Online Simulator MyEchocardiography.com

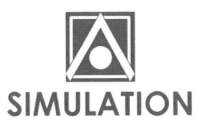

SIMULATION
ASSESSMENT OF THE PERICARDIAL EFFUSION
Echocardiography Online Simulator
MyEchocardiography.com

- Go to the link https://simulation.myechocardiography.com/
- Run Echocardiography Online Simulator using the **On/Off** Button
- Choose the patient 14 from the list **<<Patient>>** (or other patient with PE)
- From the List **<<Positions>>** Choose **Parasternal Long** or **Parasternal Short MV** or **Apical 4 Chamber** or find the position with **3D Transducer**
- Click the Button <<**Freeze**>> and Using Slider find The frame where the size of the PE is maximum.
- Click Button **<<Calculations>>** Click the Tab **<<|--|>>** Click Radio Button **<<Separation>>**
- Click the button **<<Line>>** and measure linear size of the pericardial layers separation.
- Click the button **<<Enter>>**
- Click the button << R >> to see the results.
- To change the patient, click the **On/Off** Button

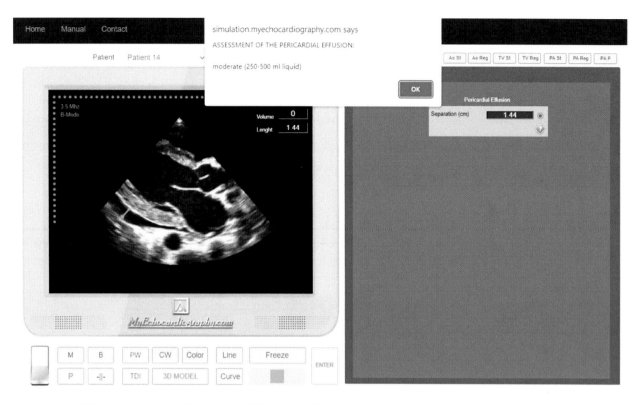

Left Parasternal View, Long axis of the Heart. Simulation By Echocardiography Online Simulator *MyEchocardiography.com*

https://www.youtube.com/watch?v=ntwsKpp3yBc

PULMONARY ARTERY

PRESSURE

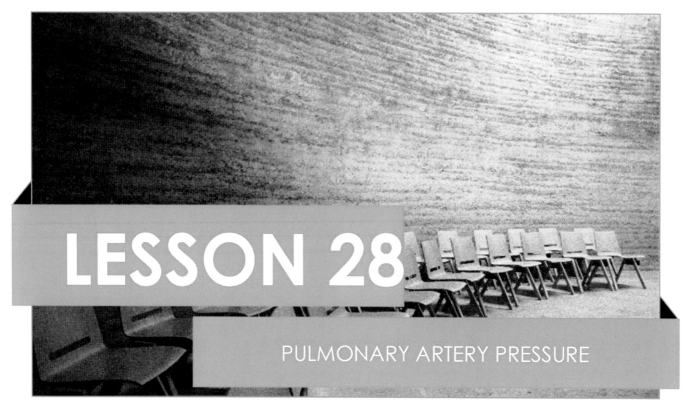

With echocardiographic examination, it is possible to determine the pulmonary artery's systolic, diastolic, and mean pressure.

PULMONARY ARTERY SYSTOLIC PRESSURE

For the assessment of pulmonary artery systolic pressure, the maximum rate of Tricuspid Regurgitation is determined and, using Bernoulli's formula, the pressure gradient between the right ventricle and the right atrium is calculated (ultrasound machines automatically calculate the pressure gradient (PG) after tracing the spectrogram by the operator). The best position is the Apical Four-Chamber.

$$\triangle p = 4V^2$$

Bernoulli's formula. V - maximum flow rate.

Tricuspid regurgitation is usual in 75-80% of the population. If the regulation signal is not optimal, echo contrast agents can be used. If there is no pulmonary artery stenosis, it can be assumed that the systolic pressure in the pulmonary artery and the right ventricle is the same. Systolic pressure in the pulmonary artery is calculated using the following formula:

$$P_{PA} = P_{RV} = PG_{TV} + P_{RA}$$

P_{PA} - Pulmonary artery systolic pressure. P_{RV} - Systolic pressure in the right ventricle. PG_{TV} - Systolic pressure gradient on the tricuspid valve (between RA and RV). P_{RA} - Pressure in the right atrium.

LESSON CONTENT

Pulmonary Artery Pressure

- Pulmonary regurgitation diagnosis.
- Degree Of Tricuspid Regurgitation By Regurgitation Jet Size (mm)
- Degree Of Tpulmonary Regurgitation By Density Of Regurgitation Jet (cw)

PULMONARY ARTERY PRESSURE

Right atrial pressure (PRA) can be measured by examining the collapse of the Inferior Vena Cava during deep inspiration (in the norm, the diameter decreases by more than 50%):

IVC diameter	Reaction on deep inhale	PRA
<15	Collapse	0-5
15-25	>50%	5-10
15-25	<50%	10-15
>25	<50%	15-20
>25 + Hepatic Vein dilatation	No reaction	>20

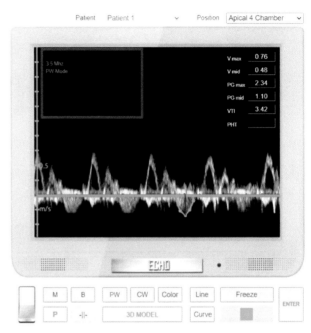

Simulator *MyEchocardiography.com*

PULMONARY ARTERY DIASTOLIC PRESSURE

For the assessment of pulmonary artery systolic pressure, the maximum rate of Pulmonary Regurgitation is determined and, using Bernoulli's formula, the pressure gradient between the pulmonary artery and the right ventricle is calculated (ultrasound machines automatically calculate the pressure gradient (PG) after tracing the spectrogram by the operator). The best position is the Parasternal View, Short axis at the level of Aorta or Pulmonary Artery.

$$\triangle p = 4V^2$$

Bernoulli's formula. V - maximum flow rate.

Pulmonary regurgitation is usual in 75-80% of the population. If the regulation signal is not optimal, echo contrast agents can be used. If there is no pulmonary artery stenosis, it can be assumed that the systolic pressure in the pulmonary artery and the right ventricle is the same.

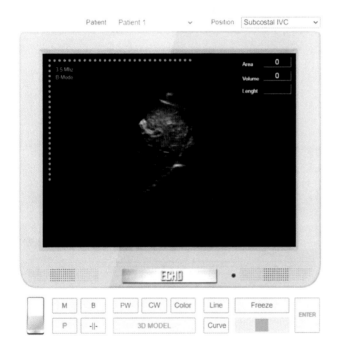

RA pressure Calculation by examining the collapse of the Inferior Vena Cava during deep inspiration. Simulation By Echocardiography Online Simulator MyEchocardiography.com

PULMONARY ARTERY PRESSURE

Systolic pressure in the pulmonary artery is calculated using the following formula:

$$P_{PA} = P_{RV} = PG_{PV} + P_{RA}$$

P_{PA} - Pulmonary artery diastolic pressure. P_{RV} - Diastolic pressure in the right ventricle. PG_{TV} - Diastolic pressure gradient on the pulmonary valve (between PA and RV). P_{RA} - Pressure in the right atrium.

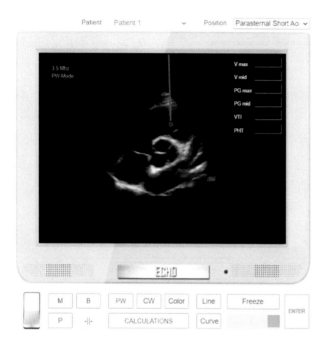

Left Parasternal View at the level of Ao valve. Control Volume Position for RVOT flow PW doppler. Simulation By Echocardiography Online Simulator MyEchocardiography.com

PULMONARY ARTERY MEAN PRESSURE

For the assessment of pulmonary artery mean pressure, the next formula is used:

Pmean = 79 - AT x 45

Pmean - Mean PA pressure. AT - RVOT Flow Acceleration Time.

Acceleration Time is The time from the opening of the valve to the peak flow. The RVOT Flow Acceleration Time AT is measured in PW mode of spectral Doppler.

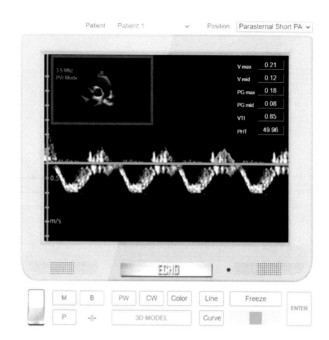

PA flow PW doppler. Calculation of PA regurgitation PG max and Pulmonary Artery Diastolic Pressure. Simulation By Echocardiography Online Simulator MyEchocardiography.com

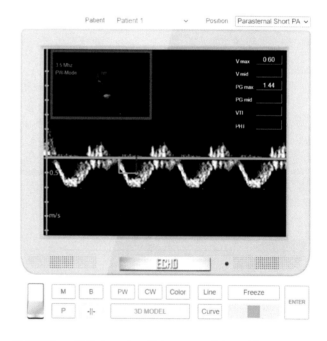

RVOT Flow PW doppler. Pulmonary Artery Mean pressure measurement by Flow Acceleration Time (AT). Simulation By Echocardiography Online Simulator MyEchocardiography.com

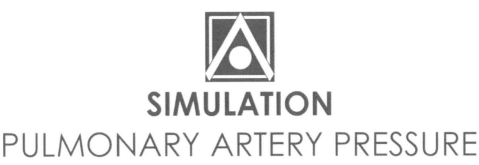

SIMULATION
PULMONARY ARTERY PRESSURE
Echocardiography Online Simulator
MyEchocardiography.com

- Go to the link https://simulation.myechocardiography.com/

- Run Echocardiography Online Simulator using the **On/Off** Button

- Choose the patient from the list **<<Patient>>**

- From the List **<<Positions>>** Choose **<<Subcostal IVC>>** (Subcostal View, Long axis of Inferior Vena Cava) or find the position with **3D Transducer**

- Examine IVC reaction on deep inhale.

- Click Button **<<Calculations>>** Click Tab **<<PA P>>**. Click the appropriate Radio Button, which corresponds to the IVC reaction in deep inhale and its size. Simulator will calculate RA pressure.

Pulmonary Artery Systolic Pressure:

- From the List **<<Positions>>** Choose <<**Apical 4 Chamber>>** (Apical 4 chamber View) or find the position with **3D Transducer**

- Click the button **<<PW>>** and place Control Volume of Pulse Wave Doppler in Tricuspid Valve.

- In the Tab Tab **<<PA P>>** click the radio Button **<<PG TV>>**

- Click the button **<<Curve>>** trace around TV regurgitation jet to measure **PG max** of tricuspid egurgitation.

- Click the button **<<Enter>>**

- Click the button **<< R >>** to see the results.

- To change the patient, click the **On/Off** Button

Pulmonary Artery Diastolic Pressure:

- From the List **<<Positions>>** Choose <<**Apical 4 Chamber>>** (Apical 4 chamber View) or find the position with **3D Transducer**

- Click the button **<<PW>>** and place Control Volume of Pulse Wave Doppler in Tricuspid Valve.

- In the Tab Tab **<<PA P>>** click the radio Button **<<PG TV>>**

- Click the button **<<Curve>>** trace around TV regurgitation jet to measure **PG max** of tricuspid egurgitation.

- Click the button **<<Enter>>**

- Click the button << R >> to see the results.
- To change the patient, click the **On/Off** Button

Pulmonary Artery Mean Pressure:

- From the List **<<Positions>>** Choose **<<Apical 4 Chamber>>** (Apical 4 chamber View) or <u>find the position</u> <u>with</u> **3D Transducer**
- Click the button **<<PW>>** and place Control Volume of Pulse Wave Doppler in Tricuspid Valve.
- In the Tab Tab **<<PA P>>** click the radio Button **<<AT>>**
- Click the button **<<Line>>** Measure time interval between start point of the **RVOT** flow and point where flow velocity starts decreasing (AT measurement).
- Click the button **<<Enter>>**
- Click the button << R >> to see the results.
- To change the patient, click the **On/Off** Button

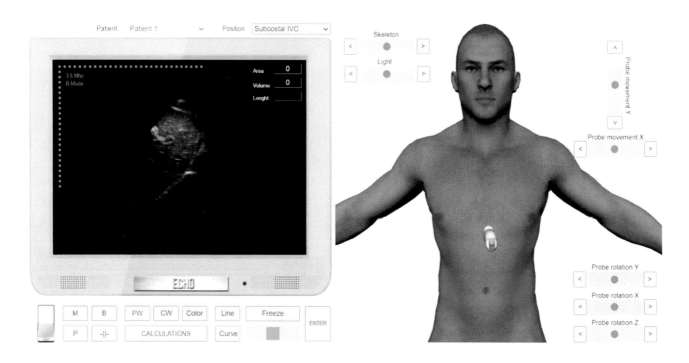

Subcostal View, the Long axis of Inferior Vena Cava. Deep inhale. Simulation By Echocardiography Online Simulator <u>MyEchocardiography.com</u>

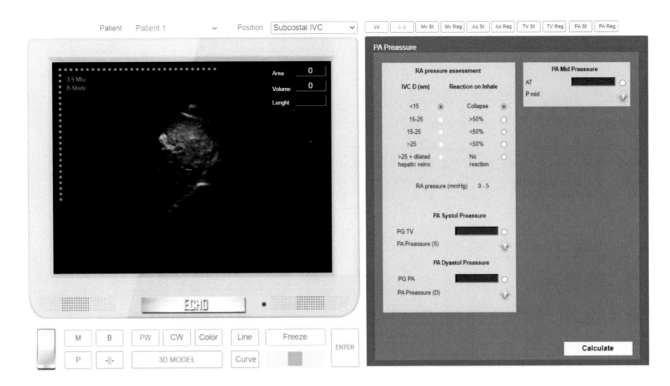

RA pressure Calculation by examining the collapse of the Inferior Vena Cava during deep inspiration. Simulation By Echocardiography Online Simulator MyEchocardiography.com

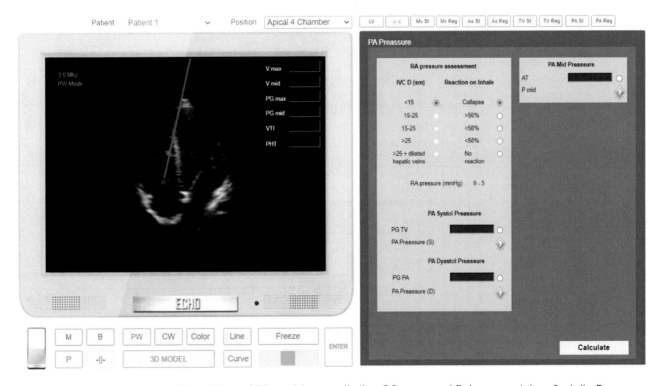

Tricuspid flow PW doppler. Calculation of Tricuspid regurgitation PG max and Pulmonary Artery Systolic Pressure. Simulation By Echocardiography Online Simulator MyEchocardiography.com

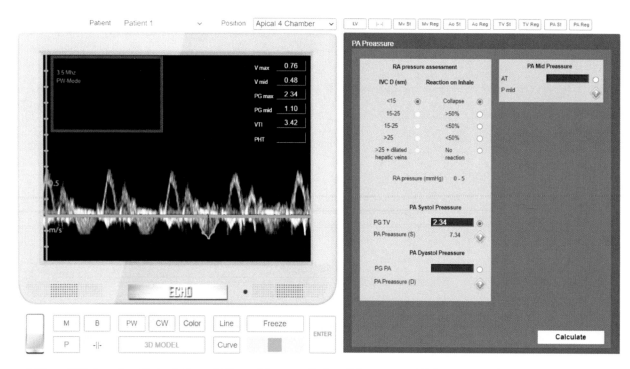

Tricuspid flow PW doppler. Calculation of Tricuspid regurgitation PG max and Pulmonary Artery Systolic Pressure.
Simulation By Echocardiography Online Simulator MyEchocardiography.com

https://youtu.be/UQO30RTZVfY

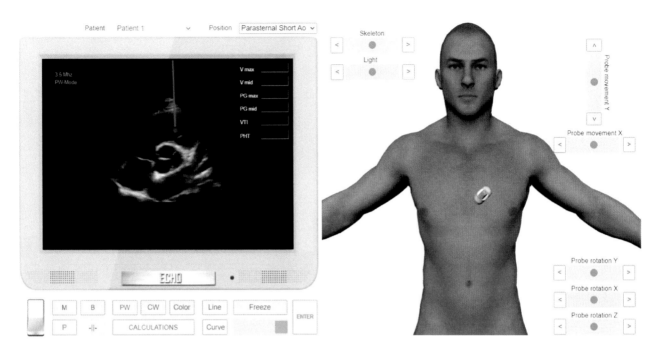

Left Parasternal View at the level of Ao valve. Control Volume Position for RVOT flow PW doppler. Simulation By Echocardiography Online Simulator MyEchocardiography.com

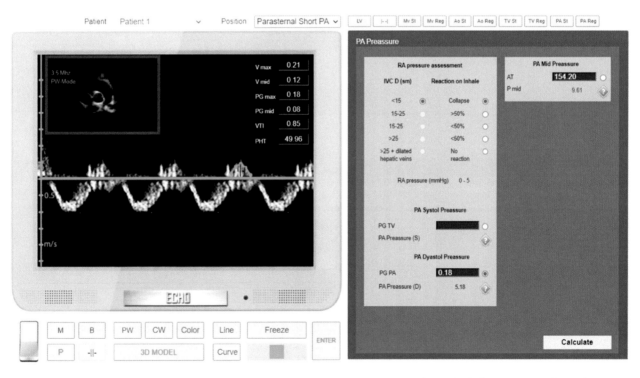

PA flow PW doppler. Calculation of PA regurgitation PG max and Pulmonary Artery Diastolic Pressure. Simulation By Echocardiography Online Simulator MyEchocardiography.com

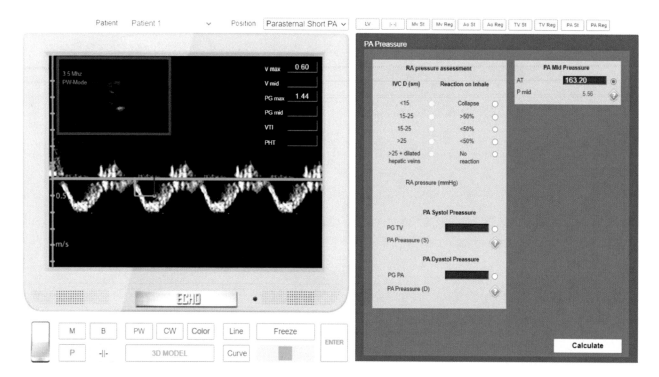

RVOT Flow PW doppler. Pulmonary Artery Mean pressure measurement by Flow Acceleration Time (AT). Simulation By Echocardiography Online Simulator MyEchocardiography.com

CARDIOMYOPATHIES

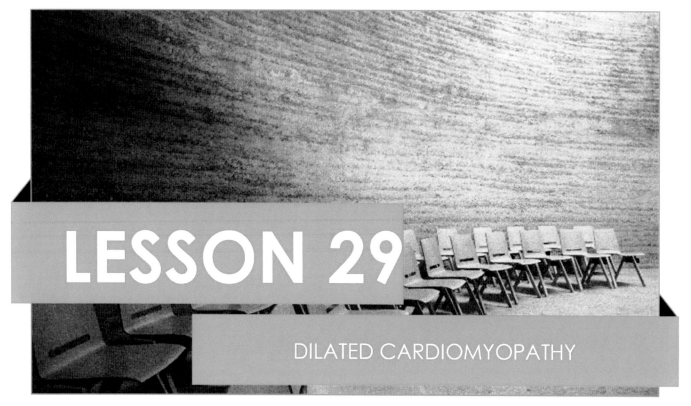

LESSON 29

DILATED CARDIOMYOPATHY

Dilated cardiomyopathy is characterized by significant dilatation of heart chambers (mainly the left ventricle) and systolic dysfunction. Despite the different etiologies, the 2D echocardiographic picture is the same in all cases. The left ventricle is spherical (linear dimensions on its short and long axis are approximately the same. The ratio is close to 1).

Quantitative values of all systolic heart function characteristics are reduced (ejection fraction <30%, stroke volume, cardiac output, etc. are reduced). There are rare cases when the dilatation is minimal, and the left ventricular dysfunction is significant.

The wall thickness of the left ventricle is mainly within the norm; in some cases, its thinning or thickening may be detected. Myocardium mass is increased in all cases. Dilatation of the chambers and fibrous rings leads to a relative deficiency of the valves (mainly mitral regurgitation. Tricuspid regurgitation is quite common). Regurgitation can be revealed by color and spectral Doppler.

Signs of left ventricular diastolic dysfunction are also not uncommon. The presence of diastolic dysfunction is a worse prognostic sign. In the dilated akinetic-hypokinetic left ventricular cavity are conditions for thrombus formation.

On the one-dimensional echocardiogram of the mitral valve, we can see increased E-point septal separation (increases the distance from the E-point to the septum. Normally, it is up to 5 mm).

DILATED CARDIOMYOPATHY

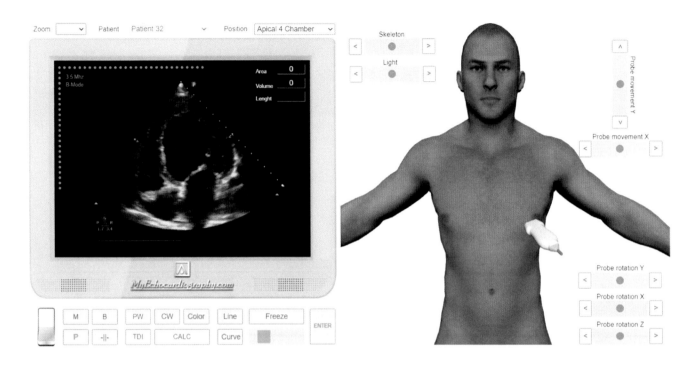

Apical 4 Chamber View. Dilated Cardiomyopathy. Simulation By Echocardiography Online Simulator MyEchocardiography.com

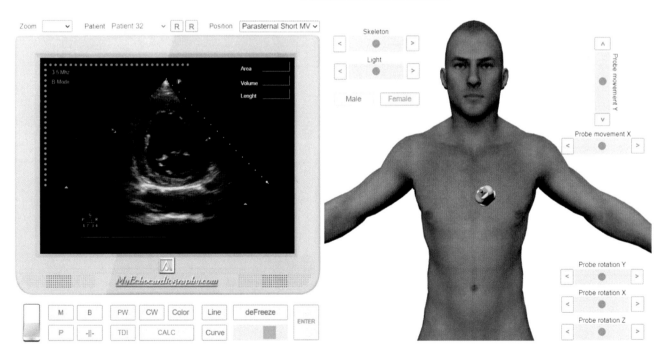

Left Parasternal View Short Axis at the Level of Mitral Valve. Dilated Cardiomyopathy. Simulation By Echocardiography Online Simulator MyEchocardiography.com

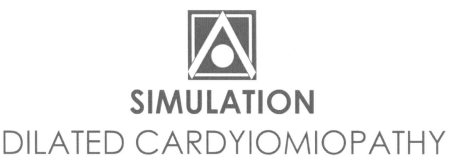

SIMULATION
DILATED CARDYIOMIOPATHY
Echocardiography Online Simulator
MyEchocardiography.com

- Go to the link https://simulation.myechocardiography.com/

- Run Echocardiography Online Simulator using the **On/Off** Button

- Choose the patient 32 from the list **<<Patient>>**

- Perform Linear and Volimetric Measurements. Calculate heart Mass. EF%. Stroke Volume. Cardiac Index.

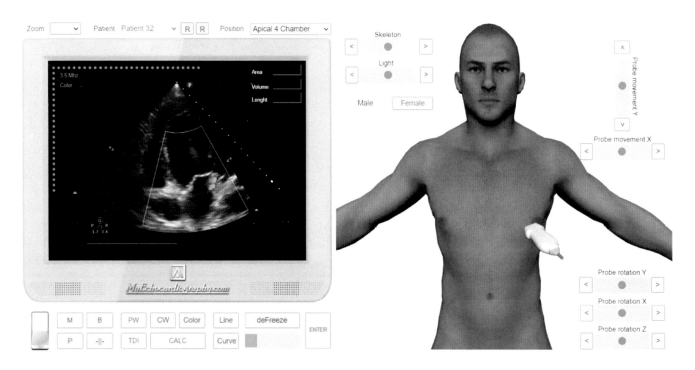

Apical 4 Chamber View. Color Doppler. Dilated Cardiomyopathy. Mild Mitral Regurgitation. Simulation By Echocardiography Online Simulator MyEchocardiography.com

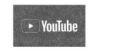

https://youtu.be/S9Bms9vxpPY

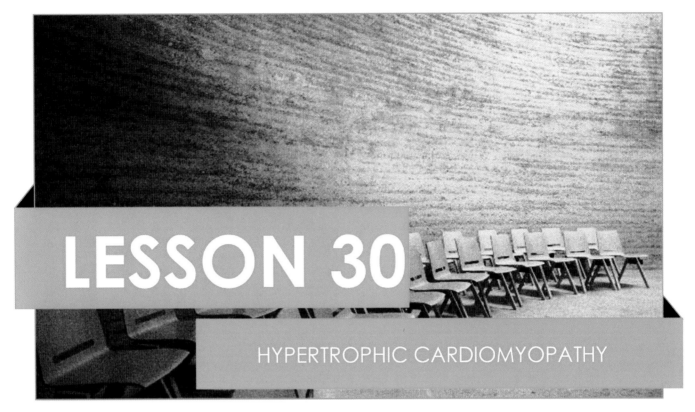

LESSON 30

HYPERTROPHIC CARDIOMYOPATHY

Hypertrophic cardiomyopathy is diagnosed when there is unexplained hypertrophy of the myocardium. Genetic changes in sarcomeres most often cause the disease. More than 50% of cases are autosomal-dominant.

Echocardiography is one of the most important methods for diagnosing hypertrophic cardiomyopathy. It detects the corresponding changes in the myocardium and excludes other possible causes of hypertrophy.

According to the nature of hypertrophy, hypertrophic cardiomyopathy can be of the following types:

- Asymmetric hypertrophy of the interventricular septum (the most frequent variant) is usually predominantly hypertrophied in its basal part.

- Symmetrical - symmetric hypertrophy of the entire left ventricle (concentric).

- Hypertrophy of the basal part of the interventricular septum (sigmoid septum).

- Hypertrophy of the apical part of the interventricular septum.

- Hypertrophy of the middle part of the ventricular cavity or papillary muscles (very rare, usually accompanied by intraventricular obstruction).

LESSON CONTENT

Hypertrophic Cardiomyopathy

- Hypertrophic Cardiomiopathy diagnosis.
- Simulation by Echocardiography Online Simulator www.MyEchocardiography.com

HYPERTROPHIC CARDIOMYOPATHY

Hypertrophic cardiomyopathy can be:

- Obstructive: systole with obstruction of the outflow tract of the left ventricle.
- Non-obstructive: without obstruction.

Hypertrophic cardiomyopathy is characterized by a Hypertrophy of the Left Ventricle, a decrease in the left ventricle volume, and dilatation of the left atrium.

Systolic function is either normal or increased. Often, the ratio of the interventricular septum's thickness to the posterior wall's thickness is greater than 1,3.

Diastolic dysfunction is noted in approximately 80% of patients.

In about a quarter of patients, the left ventricular outflow tract is narrowing. The result is its dynamic obstruction. Pre-systolic movement of the mitral valve leaflets (especially the anterior leaflet), prolongation of the leaflets, and changes in the subvalvular apparatus - contribute to the obstruction of the outflow tract. The contact point of the mitral valve cusps is located in the middle of their body, not at the ends.

A mid-systolic change in flow velocity through the aortic valve causes vibration of its leaflets, which can also be detected on a one-dimensional echocardiogram.

Spectral continuous wave Doppler is the best method for investigating dynamic obstruction. Flow velocity in the LV outflow tract is increased. It is characterized by a late peak (maximum velocity is reached at the end of systole) with a sharp lot and asymmetric character.

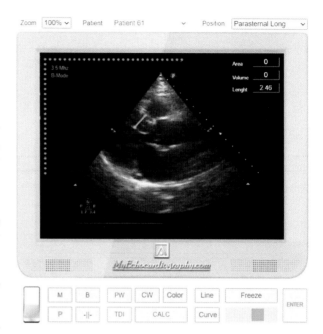

Left parasternal View, long axis. Hypertrophic Cardiomyopathy. Simulation By Echocardiography Online Simulator MyEchocardiography.com

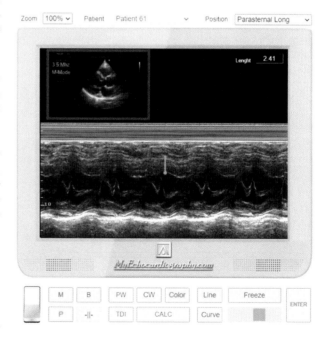

Left parasternal View, long axis. M-mode. Hypertrophic Cardiomyopathy. Simulation By Echocardiography Online Simulator MyEchocardiography.com

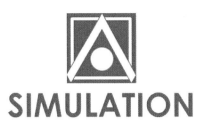

SIMULATION

HYPERTROPHIC CARDYIOMIOPATHY

Echocardiography Online Simulator
MyEchocardiography.com

- Go to the link https://simulation.myechocardiography.com/

- Run Echocardiography Online Simulator using the **On/Off** Button

- Choose the patient 61 from the list **<<Patient>>**

- Perform Linear and Volimetric Measurements. Calculate heart Mass. EF%. Stroke Volume. Cardiac Index.

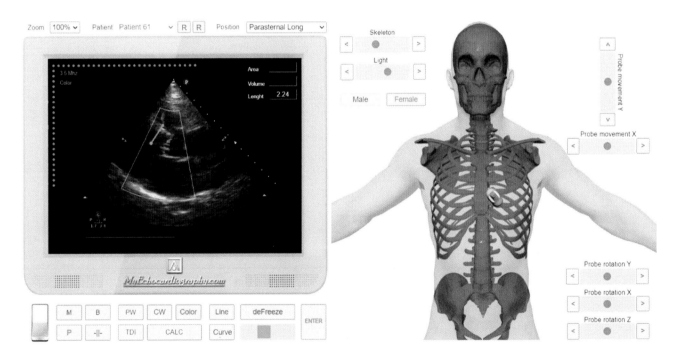

Left parasternal View, long axis. Color Doppler. Hypertrophic Cardiomyopathy. Simulation By Echocardiography Online Simulator MyEchocardiography.com

https://youtu.be/FDbKOXi2L6Q

Recommended Literature

Recommendations for the Use of Echocardiography in the Evaluation of Rheumatic Heart Disease: A Report from the American Society of Echocardiography Natesa G. Pandian at.al. Journal of the American Society of Echocardiography January 2023.

Non-Invasive Imaging in Coronary Syndromes: Recommendations of The European Association of Cardiovascular Imaging and the American Society of Echocardiography, in Collaboration with The American Society of Nuclear Cardiology, Society of Cardiovascular Computed Tomography, and Society for Cardiovascular Magnetic Resonance. Thor Edvardsen at. Al. Journal of the American Society of Echocardiography April 2022

ASE Statement on the Reintroduction of Echocardiographic Services during the COVID-19 Pandemic Judy Hung, MD, FASE (Chair), Theodore P. Abraham, MD, FASE, Meryl S. Cohen, MD, MS Ed, FASE, Michael L. Main, MD, FASE, Carol Mitchell, PhD, ACS, RDMS, RDCS, RVT, FASE, Vera H. Rigolin, MD, Journal of the American Society of Echocardiography Volume 33 Number 8. 2020.

Recommendations for Noninvasive Evaluation of Native Valvular Regurgitation A Report from the American Society of Echocardiography Developed in Collaboration with the Society for Cardiovascular Magnetic Resonance William A. Zoghbi, MD, FASE (Chair), David Adams, RCS, RDCS, FASE, Robert O. Bonow, MD, Maurice Enriquez-Sarano, MD, Elyse Foster, MD, FASE, Paul A. Grayburn, MD, FASE, Rebecca T. Hahn, MD, FASE, Yuchi Han, MD, MMSc, Judy Hung, MD, FASE, Roberto M. Lang, MD, FASE, Stephen H. Little, MD, FASE, Dipan J. Shah, MD, MMSc, Stanton Shernan, MD, FASE, Paaladinesh Thavendiranathan, MD, MSc, FASE, James D. Thomas, MD, FASE, and Neil J. Weissman, MD, FASE, Houston and Dallas, Texas; Durham, North Carolina; Chicago, Illinois; Rochester, Minnesota; San Francisco, California; New York, New York; Philadelphia, Pennsylvania; Boston, Massachusetts; Toronto, Ontario, Canada; and Washington, DC Journal of the American Society of Echocardiography April 2017.

Recommendations for the Evaluation of Left Ventricular Diastolic Function by Echocardiography: An Update from the American Society of Echocardiography and the European Association of Cardiovascular Imaging. Sherif F. Nagueh, Chair, MD, FASE,1 Otto A. Smiseth, Co-Chair, MD, PhD, Christopher P. Appleton, MD, Benjamin F. Byrd, III, MD, FASE, Hisham Dokainish, MD, FASE, Thor Edvardsen, MD, PhD, Frank A. Flachskampf, MD, PhD, FESC, Thierry C. Gillebert, MD, PhD, FESC, Allan L. Klein, MD, FASE, Patrizio Lancellotti, MD, PhD, FESC, Paolo Marino, MD, FESC, Jae K. Oh, MD. Journal of the American Society of Echocardiography April 2016.

Echocardiographic Assessment of Valve Stenosis: EAE/ASE Recommendations for Clinical Practice. Helmut Baumgartner, MD, Judy Hung, MD, Javier Bermejo, MD, PhD, John B. Chambers, MD, Arturo Evangelista, MD,† Brian P. Griffin, MD, Bernard Iung, MD, Catherine M. Otto, MD, Patricia A. Pellikka, MD, and Miguel Quiñones, MD . Journal of the American Society of Echocardiography. January 2009.

Recommendations for Cardiac Chamber Quantification by Echocardiography in Adults: An Update from the American Society of Echocardiography and the European Association of Cardiovascular Imaging. Roberto M. Lang, MD, FASE, FESC, Luigi P. Badano, MD, PhD, FESC, Victor Mor-Avi, PhD, FASE, Jonathan Afilalo, MD, MSc, Anderson Armstrong, MD, MSc, Laura Ernande, MD, PhD, Frank A. Flachskampf, MD, FESC, Elyse Foster, MD, FASE, Steven A. Goldstein, MD, Tatiana Kuznetsova, MD, PhD, Patrizio Lancellotti, MD, PhD, FESC, Denisa Muraru, MD, PhD. Journal of the American Society of Echocardiography

ACCF/AHA Task Force on Practice Guidelines. Methodology Manual and Policies From the ACCF/AHA Task Force on Practice Guidelines. American College of Cardiology Foundation and American Heart Association, Inc. cardiosource.org. 2010.

Committee on Standards for Developing Trustworthy Clinical Practice Guidelines; Institute of Medicine Clinical Practice Guidelines We Can Trust. The National Academies Press, Washington, D.C. (2013) Committee on Standards for Systematic Reviews of Comparative Effectiveness Research, Institute of Medicine Finding What Works in Health Care: Standards for Systematic Reviews. The National Academies Press, Washington, DC (2011)

Nishimura R, Otto CM, Bonow RO, et al. 2014 AHA/ACC guideline for the management of patients with valvular heart disease: a report of the American College of Cardiology/American Heart Association Task Force on Practice Guidelines. J Am Coll Cardiol In press.

Bonow RO, Carabello BA, Chatterjee K, et al. 2008 focused update incorporated into the ACC/AHA 2006 guidelines for the management of patients with valvular heart disease: a report of the American College of Cardiology/American Heart Association Task Force on Practice Guidelines (Writing Committee to revise the 1998 guidelines for the management of patients with valvular heart disease).

W.A. Zoghbi, M. Enriquez-Sarano, E. Foster, et al. Recommendations for evaluation of the severity of native valvular regurgitation with two-dimensional and Doppler echocardiography. J Am Soc Echocardiogr, 16 (2003), pp. 777-802
View PDFView articleView in ScopusGoogle Scholar.

Nagueh SF, Appleton CP, Gillebert TC, Marino PN, Oh JK, Smiseth OA, et al. Recommendations for the evaluation of left ventricular diastolic function by echocardiography. J Am Soc Echocardiogr. 2009;22:107-33.

Appleton CP. Hemodynamic determinants of Doppler pulmonary venous flow velocity components: new insights from studies in lightly sedated normal dogs. J Am Coll Cardiol 1997;30:1562-74.

Nishimura RA, Abel MD, Hatle LK, Tajik AJ. Relation of pulmonary vein to mitral flow velocities by transesophageal Doppler echocardiography. Effect of different loading conditions. Circulation 1990;81:1488-97.

Keren G, Bier A, Sherez J, Miura D, Keefe D, LeJemtel T. Atrial contraction is an important determinant of pulmonary venous flow. J Am Coll Cardiol 1986;7:693-5.

Kuecherer HF, Muhiudeen IA, Kusumoto FM, Lee E, Moulinier LE, Cahalan MK, et al. Estimation of mean left atrial pressure from transesophageal pulsed Doppler echocardiography of pulmonary venous flow. Circulation 1990;82:1127-39.

Yamamuro A, Yoshida K, Hozumi T, Akasaka T, Takagi T, Kaji S, et al. Noninvasive evaluation of pulmonary capillary wedge pressure in patients with acute myocardial infarction by deceleration time of pulmonary venous flow velocity in diastole. J Am Coll Cardiol 1999;34:

C.A. Warnes, R.G. Williams, T.M. Bashore, et al. ACC/AHA 2008 guidelines for the management of adults with congenital heart disease: a report of the American College of Cardiology/American Heart Association Task Force on Practice Guidelines (Writing Committee to Develop Guidelines on the Management of Adults With Congenital Heart Disease). Developed in Collaboration With the American Society of Echocardiography, Heart Rhythm Society, International Society for Adult Congenital Heart Disease, Society for Cardiovascular Angiography and Interventions, and Society of Thoracic Surgeons. J Am Coll Cardiol, 52 (2008), pp. e143-e263

H. Baumgartner, J. Hung, J. Bermejo, et al. Echocardiographic assessment of valve stenosis: EAE/ASE recommendations for clinical practice. Eur J Echocardiogr, 10 (2009), pp. 1-25

W.A. Zoghbi, J.B. Chambers, J.G. Dumesnil, et al. Recommendations for evaluation of prosthetic valves with echocardiography and Doppler ultrasound: a report from the American Society of Echocardiography's Guidelines and Standards Committee and the Task Force on Prosthetic Valves, developed in conjunction with the American College of Cardiology Cardiovascular Imaging Committee, Cardiac Imaging Committee of the American Heart Association, the European Association of Echocardiography, a registered branch of the European Society of Cardiology, the Japanese Society of Echocardiography and the Canadian Society of Echocardiography
J Am Soc Echocardiogr, 22 (2009), pp. 975-1014

B.J. Gersh, B.J. Maron, R.O. Bonow, et al. 2011 ACCF/AHA guideline for the diagnosis and treatment of hypertrophic cardiomyopathy: a report of the American College of Cardiology Foundation/American Heart Association Task Force on Practice Guidelines. Developed in collaboration with the American Association for Thoracic Surgery, American Society of Echocardiography, American Society of Nuclear Cardiology, Heart Failure Society of America, Heart Rhythm Society, Society for Cardiovascular Angiography and Interventions, and Society of Thoracic Surgeons
J Am Coll Cardiol, 58 (2011), pp. e212-e260

V. Regitz-Zagrosek, L.C. Blomstrom, C. Borghi, et al.
ESC guidelines on the management of cardiovascular diseases during pregnancy: the Task Force on the Management of Cardiovascular Diseases during Pregnancy of the European Society of Cardiology (ESC)
Eur Heart J, 32 (2011), pp. 3147-3197

R.P. Whitlock, J.C. Sun, S.E. Fremes, et al. Antithrombotic and thrombolytic therapy for valvular disease: antithrombotic therapy and prevention of thrombosis, 9th ed: American College of Chest Physicians Evidence-Based Clinical Practice Guidelines. Chest, 141 (2012), pp. e576S-e600S

Bonow RO, Carabello BA, Chatterjee K, de Leon CC Jr, Faxon DP, Freed MD et al. ACC/AHA 2006 guidelines for the management of patients with valvular heart disease: a report of the American College of Cardiology/American Heart Association Task Force on Practice Guidelines (writing Committee to Revise the 1998 guidelines for the management of patients with valvular heart disease) developed in collaboration with the Society of Cardiovascular Anesthesiologists endorsed by the Society for Cardiovascular Angiography and Interventions and the Society of Thoracic Surgeons. J Am Coll Cardiol 2006;48:e1-148. Table 11 Grading of pulmonary stenosis 20 Baumgartner et al Journal of the American Society of Echocardiography January 2009

Vahanian A, Baumgartner H, Bax J, Butchart E, Dion R, Filippatos G et al. Guidelines on the management of valvular heart disease: The Task Force on the Management of Valvular Heart Disease of the European Society of Cardiology. Eur Heart J 2007;28:230-68.

Chambers J, Bach D, Dumesnil J, Otto C, Shah P, Thomas J. Crossing the aortic valve in severe aortic stenosis: no longer acceptable? J Heart Valve Dis 2004;13:344-6.

Roberts WC, Ko JM. Frequency by decades of unicuspid, bicuspid, and tricuspid aortic valves in adults having isolated aortic valve replacement for aortic stenosis, with or without associated aortic regurgitation. Circulation 2005;111:920-5.

Nistri S, Sorbo MD, Marin M, Palisi M, Scognamiglio R, Thiene G. Aortic root dilatation in young men with normally functioning bicuspid aortic valves. Heart 1999;82:19-22.

Schaefer BM, Lewin MB, Stout KK, Byers PH, Otto CM. Usefulness of bicuspid aortic valve phenotype to predict elastic properties of the ascending aorta. Am J Cardiol 2007;99:686-90.

Rosenhek R, Binder T, Porenta G, Lang I, Christ G, Schemper M et al. Predictors of outcome in severe, asymptomatic aortic stenosis. N Engl J Med 2000;343:611-7. 8. Currie PJ, Seward JB, Reeder GS, Vlietstra RE, Bresnahan DR, Bresnahan JF et al. Continuous-wave Doppler echocardiographic assessment of severity of calcific aortic stenosis: a simultaneous Doppler-catheter correlative study in 100 adult patients. Circulation 1985;71: 1162-9

Smith MD, Kwan OL, DeMaria AN. Value and limitations of continuous-wave Doppler echocardiography in estimating severity of valvular stenosis. J Am Med Assoc 1986;255:3145-51.

Burwash IG, Forbes AD, Sadahiro M, Verrier ED, Pearlman AS, Thomas R et al. Echocardiographic volume flow and stenosis severity measures with changing flow rate in aortic stenosis. Am J Physiol 1993;265 (5 Pt 2):H1734-43.

Baumgartner H, Stefenelli T, Niederberger J, Schima H, Maurer G. 'Overestimation' of catheter gradients by Doppler ultrasound in patients with aortic stenosis: a predictable manifestation of pressure recovery. J Am Coll Cardiol 1999;33:1655-61.

Otto CM, Burwash IG, Legget ME, Munt BI, Fujioka M, Healy NL et al. Prospective study of asymptomatic valvular aortic stenosis. Clinical, echocardiographic, and exercise predictors of outcome. Circulation 1997;95:2262

Echocardiography Online Simulator www.myechocardiography.com

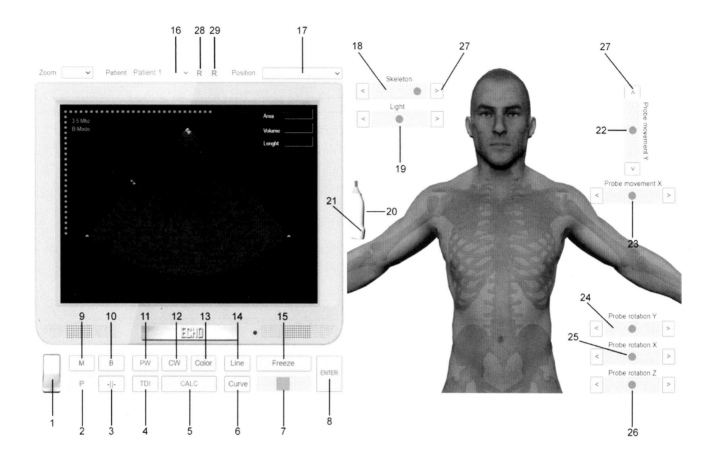

1. Turn on/off the Simulator. 2. Print. 3. Change Zoom, Gain, Contrast, Sephia. 4. Tissue Doppler. 5. Echocardiography Calculations. 6. Curve for Volume and Area measurement. 7. Change slides after freezing the image. 8. Enter Values for Calculation. 9. M-mode. 10. B-mode. 11. Pulse Wave Doppler. 12. Continuous Wave Doppler. 13. Color Doppler. 14. Line for linear measurements. 15. Freeze the image. 16. Change Patient. 17. Change Echocardiography Position. 18. Slider for show/hide sceleton. 19. Slider to increase/decrease light. 20. Transducer. 21. Transducer Marker (Pointer). 22. Slider for Probe movement in Y axis. 23. Slider for Probe movement in X axis. 24. Slider for Probe rotation around Y axis. 25. Slider for Probe tilting around Y axis. 26. Slider for Probe tilting around Z axis. 27. Slider Button. 28. Echocardiography report (User). 29. Echocardiography report (MyEchocardiography.com experts).

Made in the USA
Monee, IL
04 February 2025

1c5cc9ad-41b0-43ec-a337-ebe967c6b898R01